DIVERTICULITIS COOKBOOK

THE BEST 15 MINUTE RECIPES + 90 DAY MEAL PLAN THAT INCLUDES ALL THE FOODS YOU CAN EAT| GET BACK ENJOING LIFE BY PREVENTING FLARE-UPS AND FRUSTRATING SITUATION IN PUBLIC

Table of Contents

Introduction **8**

Chapter 1. 5Rs Method **11**

Chapter 2. Essential Shopping List **13**

Acute Phase Foods *13*

Recovery Phase Foods *13*

Prevention Foods *13*

Chapter 3. How to Deal with Symptoms **14**

How to Deal with Mild to Medium Symptoms *14*

How to Deal with Strong Symptoms *15*

Chapter 4. 90 Days Meal Plan **17**

Chapter 5. Liquid Recipes **24**

1. Apple-Cinnamon Tea *24*

2. Blueberry Green Tea *24*

3. Citrus Sports Drink *24*

4. Homemade Orange Gelatin *25*

5. Raspberry Lemonade Ice Pops *25*

6. Homemade No Pulp Orange Juice *25*

7. Apple Orange Juice *26*

8. Pineapple Mint Juice *26*

9. Celery Apple Juice *26*

10. Homemade Banana Apple Juice *27*

11. Sweet Detox Juice *27*

12. Pineapple Ginger Juice *27*

13. Carrot Orange Juice *28*

14. Strawberry Apple Juice *28*

15. Autumn Energizer Juice *28*

16. Asian Inspired Wonton Broth *29*

17. Mushroom, Cauliflower and Cabbage Broth *29*

18. Indian Inspired Vegetable Stock *30*

19. Beef Bone Broth *30*

20. Ginger, Mushroom and Cauliflower Broth *30*

21. Fish Broth *31*

22. Clear Pumpkin Broth *31*

23. Healthier Apple Juice *32*

24. Citrus Apple Juice *32*

25. Richly Fruity Juice *32*

26. Delish Grape Juice *33*

27. Lemony Grape Juice *33*

28. Holiday Special Juice *33*

29. Vitamin C Rich Juice *33*

30. Incredible Fresh Juice *34*

31. Favorite Summer Lemonade *34*

32. Ultimate Fruity Punch *34*

33. Thirst Quencher Sports Drink *35*

34. Refreshing Sports Drink *35*

35. Perfect Sunny Day Tea *36*

36. Nutritious Green Tea *36*

37. Simple Black Tea *37*

38. Lemony Black Tea *37*

39. Metabolism Booster Coffee *37*

40. Best Homemade Broth *38*

41. Clean Testing Broth *38*

42. Healing Broth *38*

43. Veggie Lover's Broth *39*

44. Brain Healthy Broth *39*

45. Minerals Rich Broth *40*

46. Holiday Favorite Gelatin *40*

47. Chicken Bone Broth *41*

48. Homemade Beef Stock *41*

49. Three-Ingredient Sugar-Free Gelatin 41
50. Cranberry-Kombucha Jell-O 42
51. Strawberry Gummies 42
52. Fruity Jell-O Stars 43
53. Sugar-Free Cinnamon Jelly 43
54. Homey Clear Chicken Broth 43
55. Oxtail Bone Broth 44
56. Chicken Bone Broth with Ginger and Lemon 44
57. Vegetable Stock 44
58. Chicken Vegetable Soup 45
59. Carrot Ginger Soup 45
60. Turkey Sweet Potato Hash 46
61. Chicken Tenders with Honey Mustard Sauce 46
62. Chicken Breasts with Cabbage and Mushrooms 47
63. Duck with Bok Choy 47
64. Beef with Mushroom and Broccoli 48
65. Beef with Zucchini Noodles 48
66. Spiced Ground Beef 49
67. Ground Beef with Veggies 49
68. Ground Beef with Greens and Tomatoes 50
69. Guacamole 50
70. Dark Chocolate with Pomegranate Seeds 51
71. Covered Bananas 51
72. Hummus with Tahini and Turmeric 51
73. Fiber Bars 52
74. Roasted Carrot Sticks in a Honey Garlic Marinade 52
75. Apple and Pistachio Salad on Spinach 52
76. Tomato Cashew Pesto 53
77. Sweet Potato Aioli 53
78. Eggplant Paste 54
79. Catalan Style Spinach 54
80. Energy Balls 54

Chapter 6. Low-Residue Recipes 56

81. Bright Red Juice 56
82. Enticing Fresh Juice 56
83. Super-Food Scramble 56
84. Family Favorite Scramble 57
85. Tasty Veggie Omelet 57
86. Garden Veggies Quiche 58
87. Stunning Breakfast Frittata 58
88. Fluffy Pumpkin Pancakes 59
89. Super-Tasty Chicken Muffins 59
90. Classic Zucchini Bread 60
91. Greek Inspired Cucumber Salad 60
92. Light Veggie Salad 60
93. Eastern European Soup 61
94. Citrus Glazed Carrots 61
95. Braised Asparagus 61
96. Spring Flavored Pasta 62
97. Versatile Mac 'n Cheese 62
98. Gluten-Free Curry 63
99. New Year's Luncheon Meal 63
100. Entertaining Wraps 64
101. Outdoor Chicken Kabobs 64
102. Flavorful Shrimp Kabobs 65
103. Pan-Seared Scallops 65
104. Mediterranean Shrimp Salad 65
105. Health Conscious People's Salad 66
106. Italian Pasta Soup 66
107. Pure Comfort Soup 67
108. Good-for-You Stew 67
109. Zero-Fiber Chicken Dish 68
110. Amazing Chicken Platter 68
111. Colorful Chicken Dinner 69

112. *Easiest Tuna Salad* 69
113. *Lemony Salmon* 70
114. *Herbed Salmon* 70
115. *Delicious Combo Dinner* 70
116. *Chicken Cutlets* 71
117. *Salsa Turkey* 71
118. *Sriracha Lime Chicken and Apple Salad* 72
119. *Pan-Seared Scallops with Lemon-Ginger Vinaigrette* 72
120. *Roasted Salmon and Asparagus* 73
121. *Orange and Maple-Glazed Salmon* 73
122. *Cod with Ginger and Black Beans* 73
123. *Halibut Curry* 74
124. *Chicken Cacciatore* 74
125. *Chicken and Bell Pepper Saute* 75
126. *Chicken Salad Sandwiches* 75
127. *Rosemary Chicken* 76
128. *Gingered Turkey Meatballs* 76

Chapter 7. Recipes With High Fiber 77

129. *Vitamins Packed Green Juice* 77
130. *Healthier Breakfast Juice* 77
131. *Summer Perfect Smoothie* 77
132. *Filling Breakfast Smoothie* 78
133. *Bright Green Breakfast Bowl* 78
134. *Quickest Breakfast Porridge* 78
135. *Halloween Morning Oatmeal* 79
136. *Authentic Bulgur Porridge* 79
137. *2-Grains Porridge* 79
138. *Savory Crepes* 80
139. *Egg-Free Omelet* 80
140. *Summer Treat Salad* 81
141. *Secretly Amazing Salad* 81
142. *Crowd-Pleasing Salad* 82
143. *South Western Salad* 82
144. *Great Luncheon Salad* 83
145. *Flavors Powerhouse Lunch Meal* 83
146. *Eye-Catching Sweet Potato Boats* 84
147. *Mexican Enchiladas* 84
148. *Unique Banana Curry* 85
149. *Vegan-Friendly Platter* 85
150. *Armenian Style Chickpeas* 86
151. *Protein-Packed Soup* 86
152. *One-Pot Dinner Soup* 87
153. *3-Beans Soup* 88
154. *Heavenly Tasty Stew* 88
155. *Thanksgiving Dinner Chili* 89
156. *Meatless Monday Chili* 89
157. *Beans Trio Chili* 90
158. *Staple Vegan Curry* 91
159. *Fragrant Vegetarian Curry* 91
160. *Omega-3 Rich Dinner Meal* 92
161. *Weekend Dinner Casserole* 93
162. *Family Dinner Pilaf* 94
163. *Meat-Free Bolognese Pasta* 94
164. *High-Fiber Dumplings* 95
165. *Pizza Made with Bamboo Fibers* 95
166. *Vegetarian Hamburgers* 96
167. *Pork Steaks with Avocado* 97
168. *Chicken with Asparagus Salad* 97
169. *Hot Pepper and Lamb Salmon* 98
170. *Pork Rolls À La Ratatouille* 99
171. *Pepper Fillet with Leek* 100
172. *Lamb Chops with Beans* 101
173. *Fillet of Beef on Spring Vegetables* 102

174. Bolognese with Zucchini Noodles *103*

175. Chicken with Chickpeas *103*

176. Ham with Chicory *104*

177. Pork Medallions With Asparagus And Coconut Curry *105*

178. Lamb with Carrot and Brussels Sprouts Spaghetti *105*

Measurement Conversion Tables.................................. 107

Conclusion 108

Introduction

What Is Diverticulitis?

Mild cases of diverticulitis are treated with antibiotics, but those suffering from severe diverticulitis may have to rest eating by mouth and may adopt a special type of diet until the bleeding and pain subside. The Diverticulitis Diet is a highly recommended diet that can help alleviate acute diverticulitis. Although this diet is supposed to be short-term, it can bring about huge relief among individuals who suffer from diverticulitis. Moreover, it can also be used by people who have a sensitive digestive system.

While the Diverticulitis Diet is designed for people who suffer from diverticulitis, people who suffer from other digestive distress can benefit from the Diverticulitis diet. Moreover, normal healthy individuals who also want to give their digestive tract enough rest can benefit from this diet.

Phases of the Diverticulitis Diet

Phase 1: Clear Fluids (During A Flare)

While going through an active flare, your symptoms can become extreme. Due to this, it's smart for you to give your bowel a period of rest. As you can imagine, the best way to do this is by sticking to a clear fluid diet. This will aid in your recovery as your body may outright reject solid foods.

It is vital to note that the clear fluid stage of the diet is NOT intended to be a long-term diet. In fact, the general expectation is that you remain in this stage for no more than a couple of days.

Please Note:

Restricting yourself to a clear fluid diet for an excessive amount of time may cause you to feel light-headed, weak, hungry, and fatigued. You can also experience muscle wasting, excessive weight loss, and depletion of vitamins and minerals.

This occurs since it's incredibly difficult to meet the body's daily caloric requirements for fat, protein, and carbohydrates through a clear fluid diet. The average person will need to provide their body with at least 200 grams of carbohydrates to have enough energy to go through the day. If you struggle with low blood sugar, diabetes, or other blood sugar challenges, you may want to monitor your blood sugar levels during this stage.

As the name implies, this phase is composed of clear liquids. These include green tea, fresh fruit juice, clear broth, and gelatin dessert. The clear liquid diet provides the body with salt, liquids, and enough nutrients to function temporarily, generally for a few days, until you can eat normal food.

Phase 2: Low-Residue/Low Fiber Diet (Immediately After A Controlled Flare)

A low-residue (or low-fiber) diet acts as the reintroduction phase, after your flare-up symptoms have mostly passed but before your body is ready for high-fiber or high residue foods.

Phase 3: High Fiber Meals (Daily Life/ Preventing Future Flares)

This final stage in the diverticulitis diet is the High Fiber diet. This stage is used to maintain a balanced diet while preventing a future flare. It is basically your general day-to-day eating routine and generally takes up the majority of your diverticulitis eating plan.

However, it is important to note that you do not want to jump directly from a significantly low fiber diet (such as a clear fluid diet) directly to a high fiber diet, as this will do more harm to your colon than good. It is always best to ease into any stage of the plan that requires an increase in your fiber intake. Aim to increase your fiber intake by 2 to 4 grams per week until you reach the recommended amount for your age and biology. Bear in mind that as you increase your fiber, you also need to increase your water intake to help move the fiber through your intestinal tract.

Causes and Symptoms

It is unclear why diverticula forms and many experts have varying opinions on the subject. For some, strains or muscle spasms, especially during bowel movements, are the key reason for pressure buildup in the colon, which pushes against the inner lining. Formerly, many experts believed that inadequate consumption of fiber, which can be found in vegetables and fruits, legumes, and grains, can result in diverticulosis. However, recent inquiries into the subject are yet to reveal any clear relationship between diverticula and the consumption of fiber-rich foods.

Another potential theory is that, although unsure of the original triggers of diverticulitis, infection tends to begin as a result of the bacteria content in stools that are pushed into the diverticula. A different theory posits that the walls of the diverticula are subject to erosions from constant and increased pressure levels in the walls of the colon.

Symptoms of Diverticulitis

Although diverticulitis isn't known to result in bothersome symptoms, people tend to report any of the following conditions:

- Constipation
- Mild abdominal cramps
- Tenderness over the affected area
- Bloating or swelling

Bear in mind that presenting with one or more of the symptoms mentioned above isn't necessarily an indication that you suffer from diverticulosis. These symptoms are quite common and present in several gastrointestinal disorders ranging from stomach ulcers to inflammatory bowel diseases to irritable bowel syndrome, gallstones, celiac disease, and appendicitis.

How Diverticulitis Is Diagnosed

Since symptoms of diverticulitis do not readily present in many people, the condition is usually discovered when the patient is being screened for polyps or evaluated for other conditions. Gastroenterologists can easily locate and reveal diverticula in the colon using a procedure requiring a tiny camera attached to the end of a lighted, flexible tube inserted into the rectum. Another procedure that can be used is sigmoidoscopy in which a short tube is used to probe the lower areas of the colon and the rectum alone. For colonoscopy procedures, a longer tube is used, and the whole colon is examined. However, the discovery of diverticulosis isn't limited to gastrointestinal procedures alone and can also be discovered via imaging tests such as barium x-rays and computer tomography (CT) scans.

How Is Diverticulitis Treated?

When diverticula develops on the colon, they don't tend to occur on their own. For most patients, the symptoms are never present, and no treatments are necessary. However, when the condition is accompanied by symptoms, such as constipation, bloating, bleeding, and abdominal pain, your doctor could place you on a diet with high fiber content. The choice of diet is meant to soften stools and make them easier to pass. According to daily requirements, it's advised that we consume about 20 to 35 grams of fiber, even though many people only ever consume about half of the said amount daily.

The easiest method of improving fiber intake is to consume more grains, vegetables, and fruits. Some examples of foods with high, healthy fiber content include lima beans, broccoli, apples, squash, kidney beans, pears, and baked beans. Alternatively, your doctor could recommend fiber supplements such as polycarbophil, methylcellulose, or psyllium. These products tend to come in different forms like wafers, powders, or pills. Supplemental fiber products work like high-fiber foods, helping to soften and bulk up stool, making bowel movements easier and less strenuous. Your doctor could also prescribe some medication to reduce the level of colon spasms, which can result in discomfort and abdominal cramping.

Chapter 1. 5Rs Method

In this section, we're going to cover diverticulitis flare-ups, specifically how to manage them, how to reduce the duration of a flare-up, and how to prevent them. This method is divided into 5 steps, which we will call 5Rs, there are natural remedies and actions that you can take and easily add to your answer in your daily life.

So back to the first step, how to recognize a flare-up:

This is important because sometimes when your body is telling you something is wrong, something's going on we have such busy lives that we ignore those signals so sometimes you feel a little bit of pain or a little bit of discomfort, or even before a flare you may recognize that you're more tired than you usually are and these signs come before a full-blown flare up and I want you to practice listening to your body and recognizing these signs before the flare-up becomes more severe it's important to recognize the flare-up right away so that you can begin your healing process as soon as possible. So even after that step, you want anything adding to the problem you want to eat an anti-inflammatory diet you want to drink mineral-rich mineral-rich water you want to drink green teas herbal teas aloe vera juice drinks that reduce inflammation and help clean your tissues you also want to reduce movement so while you're healing you want to be resting laying down make sure you're not working out those days or anything to add stress to the body speak stress you also want to reduce any emotional stressors as much as possible so if you're a very busy person and you're at work you know always on the go and you use dealing with a lot of stress try to minimize that during the flare because your body needs all things you can get to heal and actually emotional stress is very draining. The next step is repairs, so repair means you know your issue and your tests in the wall have been damaged, it's been infected it's inflamed, so of course, you need to do something to repair the damage. The antibiotics may be got rid of the infection it doesn't get rid of any damage done by the infection so you always want to keep that in mind and repair consists of some things already mentioned such as your anti-inflammatory beverages like aloe vera and your mineral water but add to that bone broth which is very anti-inflammatory full of nutrients very healing and also look at what you're eating. Eat foods that are easier to digest than do not stress out your bowels so you might have soups that are more brothy than they are full of you know veggies and definitely no meat so this is your repair process. Also in the repair process, there are a few things you want to look out for minimizing the number of different foods as you eat especially when you're thinking about one meal you know one be eating five different types of food. You'll need rice, chicken, broccoli, onions, and garlic because when you're sick and you're trying to heal the more work you're put on your digestive system the longer it will take to heal so don't interfere with your healing try to eat simply. Foods: If you feel like you can go back to vegetables eat steamed vegetables. So the next step is removed, so remove is after the flare-up, after you've healed. After you turn back to work and you feel good, you're not experiencing pains, chills, or fever now you get to the removal step. Your liquid diet and your soft foods have helped your body heal but now is the time since your intestines are in a less sensitive space. Now is the time to do a heavier cleanse of your bowels this is when you increase your fiber intake, what you want to do is add bentonite clay or activated charcoal.

Fiber helps your intestines push stool through the body but that clay in the charcoal but that helps with is drawing the waste that has been building up in your mucosal layers out and to move out all that waste that was built up in the diverticula and you want to do this in combination with certain herbs so there are key herbs for anybody experiencing inflammation in the gut so in combination with the fiber the midnight clay and activated charcoal. Renourish: After your body's gone through all this stress and flare-ups you may have depletes your body of some nutrients during that time and you want to replenish those nutrients so increase your vitamin intake your antioxidants like your vitamin C. Make sure you always have a multivitamin and take those every day, increase your mineral intake people are usually deficient in magnesium and calcium and especially when your body is undergoing stress the first nutrients that get used up are usually minerals and so to have a good supplement with all your minerals. Start the repair process by consuming anti-inflammatory liquids and foods to remove that stool in those wastes from the bowels and renourish replenish your minerals and replenish your vitamin.

Chapter 2. Essential Shopping List

A diet food list for diverticular diseases with several decades of fiber-rich foods, clear liquid foods, and low-fiber foods helps people with diverticulitis know what's safe to eat at any one time. The foods are categorized into three, namely:

Acute Phase Foods

This category comprises foods for a clear liquid diet:

- Dry toast
- Jell-O without fruit
- Fruit juices without pulp
- Plain saltine crackers
- Chicken or beef broth
- Water, tea, or coffee (without dairy)
- Popsicles or ice chips (pulp-free)

Recovery Phase Foods

This category includes foods for a low-fiber diet:

- Yogurt
- Toast and soft or hard-boiled eggs
- Well cooked vegetables (skinned)
- Vegetable soup
- Low-fiber cereals
- Canned fruits (pulp-free), Juices (pulp-free)
- Peanut butter
- Macaroni, rice, and plain noodles
- Fish, meat, and poultry

Prevention Foods

This category is for reintroducing fiber into your diet:

- Fish, poultry, meat
- Wild rice
- Brown rice
- Vegetables
- Fruits with pulp
- Cereals and bread (whole grain variety)
- Dried beans and lentils
- All foods with low-FODMAP

Chapter 3. How to Deal with Symptoms

Patients may have various scenes of Diverticular disease or diverticulitis, and it might be hard to recognize the two. Milder scenes of torment might be dealt with at home with bed rest, prescriptions for torment and fit, and an unmistakable fluid diet. Patients ought to take their temperature as often as possible and push on their lower left guts where most Diverticular are found.

At the principal indication of fever or expanding delicacy—indications of aggravation—a specialist ought to be counseled instantly for a conceivable visit to his office and/or the start of anti-infection agents; there is nothing as profitable as a physical examination by the specialist to settle on choices about further treatment or hospitalization.

How to Deal with Mild to Medium Symptoms

Most patients with Diverticulosis have negligible or no symptoms and don't require particular treatment. A typical fiber diet is fitting to counteract blockage and maybe keep the arrangement more Diverticular.

Patients with gentle symptoms of stomach pain because of strong fit in the range of the Diverticular may profit by hostile to uncontrollable medications, for example:

- Hyoscyamine (Levsin)
- Phenobarbital (Donnatal)
- Chlordiazepoxide (Librax)
- Dicyclomine (Bentyl)
- Scopolamine
- Atropine

At the point when diverticulitis happens, anti-toxins, for the most pa2rt are required. Oral anti-infection agents are adequate when symptoms are gentle.

A few cases of normally recommended anti-microbials include:

- Flagyl (metronidazole)
- Cipro (Ciprofloxacin)
- Keflex (Cephalexin)
- Vibramycin (doxycycline)

What are different medications for diverticulitis?

Fluid or low fiber foods are informed during intense attacks concerning diverticulitis. This is done to decrease the measure of material that goes through the colon, which in any event hypothetically, may irritate the diverticulitis. In extreme diverticulitis, where patients suffer from intense pain and high fever, the patients are often hospitalized to be treated with intravenous anti-infection agents. Surgery is required for patients with steady entrails obstacles, bleeding, or sore not reacting to antibiotics.

How to Deal with Strong Symptoms

Diverticulitis that does not react to restorative treatment requires surgical mediation. Surgery normally includes drainage of any collections of discharge and resection (surgical evacuation) of the portion of the colon containing the Diverticular, as a rule, the sigmoid colon. Surgical expulsion of the bleeding diverticulum likewise is important for those with determined bleeding. In patients requiring surgery to stop industrious bleeding, it is important to decide precisely where the bleeding originates from, keeping in mind the end goal to direct the specialist.

Now and then, Diverticular can disintegrate into the nearby urinary bladder, creating serious intermittent pee contamination and entry of gas amid pee. This circumstance additionally requires surgery.

Now and then, surgery might be proposed for patients with regular, repetitive attacks of diverticulitis, prompting different courses of anti-toxins, hospitalizations, and days lost from work. During surgery, the objective is to evacuate all or all of the colon containing Diverticular to anticipate future diverticulitis occurrences.

Chapter 4. 90 Days Meal Plan

DAY	BREAKFAST	LUNCH	DINNER	SNACK
1	Apple-Cinnamon Tea	Asian Inspired Wonton Broth	Beef Bone Broth	Raspberry Lemonade Ice Pops
2	Blueberry Green Tea	Mushroom, Cauliflower and Cabbage Broth	Indian Inspired Vegetable Stock	Three-Ingredient Sugar-Free Gelatin
3	Homemade No Pulp Orange Juice	Ginger, Mushroom and Cauliflower Broth	Fish Broth	Cranberry-Kombucha Jell-O
4	Homemade Banana Apple Juice	Clear Pumpkin Broth	Best Homemade Broth	Sugar-Free Cinnamon Jelly
5	Strawberry Apple Juice	Clean Testing Broth	Veggie Lover's Broth	Raspberry Lemonade Ice Pops
6	Celery Apple Juice	Vegetable Stock	Chicken Bone Broth with Ginger and Lemon	Three-Ingredient Sugar-Free Gelatin
7	Autumn Energizer Juice	Carrot Ginger Soup	Chicken Vegetable Soup	Cranberry-Kombucha Jell-O
8	Super-Food Scramble	Light Veggie Salad	Herbed Salmon	Mediterranean Shrimp Salad
9	Tasty Veggie Omelet	Spring Flavored Pasta	Chicken Cutlets	Health Conscious People's Salad
10	Garden Veggies Quiche	Entertaining Wraps	Sriracha Lime Chicken and Apple Salad	Citrus Glazed Carrots
11	Stunning Breakfast Frittata	Zero-Fiber Chicken Dish	Halibut Curry	Classic Zucchini Bread

12	Greek Inspired Cucumber Salad	Lemony Salmon	Rosemary Chicken	Chicken Salad Sandwiches
13	Classic Zucchini Bread	Cod with Ginger and Black Beans	Delicious Combo Dinner	Gingered Turkey Meatballs
14	Super-Tasty Chicken Muffins	Flavorful Shrimp Kabobs	Gluten-Free Curry	Outdoor Chicken Kabobs
15	Healthier Breakfast Juice	Flavors Powerhouse Lunch Meal	Chicken with Chickpeas	Good-for-You Chocolate Chip Cookies
16	Bright Green Breakfast Bowl	Great Luncheon Salad	Lamb Chops with Beans	Oatmeal Sunflower Bread
17	Filling Breakfast Smoothie	Mexican Enchiladas	Fillet of Beef on Spring Vegetables	Oat and Wheat Cookies
18	Authentic Bulgur Porridge	Vegan-Friendly Platter	Bolognese with Zucchini Noodles	Maple Oatmeal Bread
19	Egg-Free Omelet	Fragrant Vegetarian Curry	Pork Medallions With Asparagus And Coconut Curry	Oatmeal Spice Cookies
20	Savory Crepes	Cabbage Wrap	Lamb with Carrot and Brussels Sprouts Spaghetti	German Dark Bread
21	Vitamins Packed Green Juice	Veal with Asparagus	Salmon with Sesame Seeds and Mushrooms	Trail Mix Cookies
22	2-Grains Porridge	Stuffed Trout with Mushrooms	One-Pot Dinner Soup	Oatmeal Sunflower Bread
23	Summer Perfect Smoothie	Salmon with Basil and Avocado	Unique Banana Curry	White Chocolate-Cranberry Cookies
24	Quickest Breakfast Porridge	Vegetarian Hamburgers	Secretly Amazing Salad	Maple Oatmeal Bread
25	Halloween Morning Oatmeal	Beans Trio Chili	Weekend Dinner Casserole	German Dark Bread

26	Healthier Breakfast Juice	Crowd-Pleasing Salad	Family Dinner Pilaf	Good-for-You Chocolate Chip Cookies
27	Bright Green Breakfast Bowl	Meat-Free Bolognese Pasta	3-Beans Soup	Oat and Wheat Cookies
28	Filling Breakfast Smoothie	Pepper Fillet with Leek	Pork Steaks with Avocado	White Chocolate-Cranberry Cookies
29	Healthier Breakfast Juice	Flavors Powerhouse Lunch Meal	Chicken with Chickpeas	Good-for-You Chocolate Chip Cookies
30	Bright Green Breakfast Bowl	Great Luncheon Salad	Lamb Chops with Beans	Oatmeal Sunflower Bread
31	Filling Breakfast Smoothie	Mexican Enchiladas	Fillet of Beef on Spring Vegetables	Oat and Wheat Cookies
32	Authentic Bulgur Porridge	Vegan-Friendly Platter	Bolognese with Zucchini Noodles	Maple Oatmeal Bread
33	Egg-Free Omelet	Fragrant Vegetarian Curry	Pork Medallions With Asparagus And Coconut Curry	Oatmeal Spice Cookies
34	Savory Crepes	Cabbage Wrap	Lamb with Carrot and Brussels Sprouts Spaghetti	German Dark Bread
35	Vitamins Packed Green Juice	Veal with Asparagus	Salmon with Sesame Seeds and Mushrooms	Trail Mix Cookies
36	2-Grains Porridge	Stuffed Trout with Mushrooms	One-Pot Dinner Soup	Oatmeal Sunflower Bread
37	Summer Perfect Smoothie	Salmon with Basil and Avocado	Unique Banana Curry	White Chocolate-Cranberry Cookies
38	Quickest Breakfast Porridge	Vegetarian Hamburgers	Secretly Amazing Salad	Maple Oatmeal Bread
39	Halloween Morning Oatmeal	Beans Trio Chili	Weekend Dinner Casserole	German Dark Bread

40	Healthier Breakfast Juice	Crowd-Pleasing Salad	Family Dinner Pilaf	Good-for-You Chocolate Chip Cookies
41	Bright Green Breakfast Bowl	Meat-Free Bolognese Pasta	3-Beans Soup	Oat and Wheat Cookies
42	Filling Breakfast Smoothie	Pepper Fillet with Leek	Pork Steaks with Avocado	White Chocolate-Cranberry Cookies
43	Healthier Breakfast Juice	Flavors Powerhouse Lunch Meal	Chicken with Chickpeas	Good-for-You Chocolate Chip Cookies
44	Bright Green Breakfast Bowl	Great Luncheon Salad	Lamb Chops with Beans	Oatmeal Sunflower Bread
45	Filling Breakfast Smoothie	Mexican Enchiladas	Fillet of Beef on Spring Vegetables	Oat and Wheat Cookies
46	Authentic Bulgur Porridge	Vegan-Friendly Platter	Bolognese with Zucchini Noodles	Maple Oatmeal Bread
47	Egg-Free Omelet	Fragrant Vegetarian Curry	Pork Medallions With Asparagus And Coconut Curry	Oatmeal Spice Cookies
48	Savory Crepes	Cabbage Wrap	Lamb with Carrot and Brussels Sprouts Spaghetti	German Dark Bread
49	Vitamins Packed Green Juice	Veal with Asparagus	Salmon with Sesame Seeds and Mushrooms	Trail Mix Cookies
50	2-Grains Porridge	Stuffed Trout with Mushrooms	One-Pot Dinner Soup	Oatmeal Sunflower Bread
51	Summer Perfect Smoothie	Salmon with Basil and Avocado	Unique Banana Curry	White Chocolate-Cranberry Cookies
52	Quickest Breakfast Porridge	Vegetarian Hamburgers	Secretly Amazing Salad	Maple Oatmeal Bread
53	Halloween Morning Oatmeal	Beans Trio Chili	Weekend Dinner Casserole	German Dark Bread

54	Healthier Breakfast Juice	Crowd-Pleasing Salad	Family Dinner Pilaf	Good-for-You Chocolate Chip Cookies
55	Bright Green Breakfast Bowl	Meat-Free Bolognese Pasta	3-Beans Soup	Oat and Wheat Cookies
56	Filling Breakfast Smoothie	Pepper Fillet with Leek	Pork Steaks with Avocado	White Chocolate-Cranberry Cookies
57	Healthier Breakfast Juice	Flavors Powerhouse Lunch Meal	Chicken with Chickpeas	Good-for-You Chocolate Chip Cookies
58	Bright Green Breakfast Bowl	Great Luncheon Salad	Lamb Chops with Beans	Oatmeal Sunflower Bread
59	Filling Breakfast Smoothie	Mexican Enchiladas	Fillet of Beef on Spring Vegetables	Oat and Wheat Cookies
60	Authentic Bulgur Porridge	Vegan-Friendly Platter	Bolognese with Zucchini Noodles	Maple Oatmeal Bread
61	Egg-Free Omelet	Fragrant Vegetarian Curry	Pork Medallions With Asparagus And Coconut Curry	Oatmeal Spice Cookies
62	Savory Crepes	Cabbage Wrap	Lamb with Carrot and Brussels Sprouts Spaghetti	German Dark Bread
63	Vitamins Packed Green Juice	Veal with Asparagus	Salmon with Sesame Seeds and Mushrooms	Trail Mix Cookies
64	2-Grains Porridge	Stuffed Trout with Mushrooms	One-Pot Dinner Soup	Oatmeal Sunflower Bread
65	Summer Perfect Smoothie	Salmon with Basil and Avocado	Unique Banana Curry	White Chocolate-Cranberry Cookies
66	Quickest Breakfast Porridge	Vegetarian Hamburgers	Secretly Amazing Salad	Maple Oatmeal Bread
67	Halloween Morning Oatmeal	Beans Trio Chili	Weekend Dinner Casserole	German Dark Bread

68	Healthier Breakfast Juice	Crowd-Pleasing Salad	Family Dinner Pilaf	Good-for-You Chocolate Chip Cookies
69	Bright Green Breakfast Bowl	Meat-Free Bolognese Pasta	3-Beans Soup	Oat and Wheat Cookies
70	Filling Breakfast Smoothie	Pepper Fillet with Leek	Pork Steaks with Avocado	White Chocolate-Cranberry Cookies
71	Healthier Breakfast Juice	Flavors Powerhouse Lunch Meal	Chicken with Chickpeas	Good-for-You Chocolate Chip Cookies
72	Bright Green Breakfast Bowl	Great Luncheon Salad	Lamb Chops with Beans	Oatmeal Sunflower Bread
73	Filling Breakfast Smoothie	Mexican Enchiladas	Fillet of Beef on Spring Vegetables	Oat and Wheat Cookies
74	Authentic Bulgur Porridge	Vegan-Friendly Platter	Bolognese with Zucchini Noodles	Maple Oatmeal Bread
75	Egg-Free Omelet	Fragrant Vegetarian Curry	Pork Medallions With Asparagus And Coconut Curry	Oatmeal Spice Cookies
76	Savory Crepes	Cabbage Wrap	Lamb with Carrot and Brussels Sprouts Spaghetti	German Dark Bread
77	Vitamins Packed Green Juice	Veal with Asparagus	Salmon with Sesame Seeds and Mushrooms	Trail Mix Cookies
78	2-Grains Porridge	Stuffed Trout with Mushrooms	One-Pot Dinner Soup	Oatmeal Sunflower Bread
79	Summer Perfect Smoothie	Salmon with Basil and Avocado	Unique Banana Curry	White Chocolate-Cranberry Cookies
80	Quickest Breakfast Porridge	Vegetarian Hamburgers	Secretly Amazing Salad	Maple Oatmeal Bread
81	Halloween Morning Oatmeal	Beans Trio Chili	Weekend Dinner Casserole	German Dark Bread

82	Healthier Breakfast Juice	Crowd-Pleasing Salad	Family Dinner Pilaf	Good-for-You Chocolate Chip Cookies
83	Bright Green Breakfast Bowl	Meat-Free Bolognese Pasta	3-Beans Soup	Oat and Wheat Cookies
84	Filling Breakfast Smoothie	Pepper Fillet with Leek	Pork Steaks with Avocado	White Chocolate-Cranberry Cookies
85	Healthier Breakfast Juice	Flavors Powerhouse Lunch Meal	Chicken with Chickpeas	Good-for-You Chocolate Chip Cookies
86	Bright Green Breakfast Bowl	Great Luncheon Salad	Lamb Chops with Beans	Oatmeal Sunflower Bread
87	Filling Breakfast Smoothie	Mexican Enchiladas	Fillet of Beef on Spring Vegetables	Oat and Wheat Cookies
88	Authentic Bulgur Porridge	Vegan-Friendly Platter	Bolognese with Zucchini Noodles	Maple Oatmeal Bread
89	Egg-Free Omelet	Fragrant Vegetarian Curry	Pork Medallions With Asparagus And Coconut Curry	Oatmeal Spice Cookies
90	Savory Crepes	Cabbage Wrap	Lamb with Carrot and Brussels Sprouts Spaghetti	German Dark Bread

Chapter 5. Liquid Recipes

1. Apple-Cinnamon Tea

Preparation Time: 5 minutes

Cooking Time: 15 minutes

Servings: 4

Ingredients:

- 1 cup chopped apples, Honey Crisp, Fuji, Granny Smith, or Gala
- 3 cinnamon sticks
- 1-quart water
- 2 bags Earl Grey tea (caffeinated or decaffeinated)
- 1/3 cup honey, plus more if desired

Directions:

1. In a large saucepan over high heat, set the apples, cinnamon sticks, and water. Bring to a boil. Set the heat to medium and stir for 15 minutes.
2. Remove from the heat and add the Earl Grey teabags. Steep for 10 minutes.
3. Using a slotted spoon, detach the tea bags, apples, and cinnamon sticks. Attach the honey and stir until it dissolves. Taste and add more honey, if desired. Serve hot.

Nutrition:

- Calories: 101 kcal
- Fat: 1 g
- Carbs: 27 g
- Fiber: 1 g
- Protein: 1 g
- Sodium: 6 mg

2. Blueberry Green Tea

Preparation Time: 5 minutes

Cooking Time: 5 minutes

Servings: 4

Ingredients:

- 1/2 cup fresh or frozen blueberries
- 1-quart water
- 2 bags green tea (caffeinated or decaffeinated)
- 1/3 cup honey, plus more if desired

Directions:

1. In a saucepan over high heat, place the blueberries and water and bring to a boil. Set the heat to low and stir for 5 minutes.
2. Detach from the heat and add the green tea bags. Steep for 10 minutes.
3. Using a slotted spoon, set the tea bags and blueberries. Attach the honey and stir until it dissolves. Taste and add more honey, if desired. Serve hot.

Nutrition:

- Calories: 95 kcal
- Fat: 0 g
- Carbs: 26 g
- Fiber: 1 g
- Protein: 1 g
- Sodium: 7 mg

3. Citrus Sports Drink

Preparation Time: 5 minutes

Cooking Time: 0 minutes

Servings: 8

Ingredients:

- 4 cups coconut water
- 4 large oranges juice (about 1 ½ cup), strained
- 2 tbsp. lemon juice, strained
- 2 tbsp. honey or maple syrup
- 1 tsp. sea salt

Directions:

1. Place the coconut water, orange juice, lemon juice, honey, and salt in a jug or pitcher.
2. Stir until the salt is dissolved.
3. Serve cold.

Nutrition:

- Calories: 59 kcal
- Fat: 1 g
- Carbs: 14 g
- Fiber: 1 g
- Protein: 1 g
- Sodium: 304 mg

4. Homemade Orange Gelatin

Preparation Time: 4 hours 10 minutes

Cooking Time: 3 minutes

Servings: 4

Ingredients:

- 8 large oranges juice (about 3 cups), strained and divided
- 2 tbsp. unflavored gelatin
- 2 tbsp. honey or maple syrup

Directions:

1. In a large bowl, pour in 1/2 cup of orange juice and sprinkle with gelatin. Whisk well and let sit until the gelatin begins to set but is not quite smooth.
2. In a saucepan over low heat, pour in the remaining 2 ½ cups of orange juice and cook until just before boiling, 2–3 minutes.
3. Remove from the heat and pour the hot juice into the gelatin mixture. Attach the honey or maple syrup and stir until the gelatin is dissolved.
4. Pour into an 8 x 8 inches baking dish and transfer to the refrigerator.
5. Cool for 4 hours to set. Serve cold.

Nutrition:

- Calories: 127 kcal
- Fat: 1 g
- Carbs: 28 g
- Fiber: 1 g
- Protein: 6 g
- Sodium: 2 mg

5. Raspberry Lemonade Ice Pops

Preparation Time: 4 hours 10 minutes

Cooking Time: 0 minutes

Servings: 4 Ice pops

Ingredients:

- 3 cups frozen raspberries
- 1 tsp. lemon juice, strained
- 1/4 cup coconut water
- 1/4 cup honey or maple syrup

Directions:

1. In a blender, puree the raspberries, lemon juice, and coconut water until smooth.
2. Set the mixture through a fine-mesh strainer into a bowl to remove the seeds. Stir in the honey until well mixed.
3. Divide the mixture equally among 4 popsicle molds and freeze until solid, 3–4 hours.

Nutrition:

- Calories: 120 kcal
- Fat: 0 g
- Carbs: 31 g
- Fiber: 7 g
- Protein: 2 g
- Sodium: 2 mg

6. Homemade No Pulp Orange Juice

Preparation Time: 5 minutes

Cooking Time: 0 minutes

Servings: 1 ½ cup

Ingredients:

- 4 Oranges

Directions:

1. Lightly squeeze the oranges on a hard surface to soften the exterior. Slice each in half.

2. Squeeze each orange over a fine-mesh strainer.
3. Gently, press the pulp to extract all possible liquid.
4. Serve over ice. Enjoy!

Nutrition:

- Calories: 50 kcal
- Fat: 0.2 g
- Carbs: 11.5 g
- Protein: 0.8 g

7. Apple Orange Juice

Preparation Time: 5 minutes

Cooking Time: 0 minutes

Servings: 2

Ingredients:

- 1 Gala apple, peeled, cored, and sliced
- 2 oranges, peeled, halved, and seeded
- 2 tsp. honey (optional)
- 3/4 cup water

Directions:

1. Squeeze each orange over a fine-mesh strainer.
2. Gently, press the pulp to extract as much liquid as possible.
3. Add in the apple, water, and orange juice in your blender and pulse.
4. Set a fine-mesh strainer in a bowl. Before transferring your juice into the strainer.
5. Once again, gently press the pulp to remove all possible liquid, then discard it.
6. Stir in your honey, then serve over ice.

Nutrition:

- Calories: 180 kcal
- Fat: 1 g
- Carbs: 43 g
- Fiber: 1 g
- Protein: 2 g

8. Pineapple Mint Juice

Preparation Time: 5 minutes.

Cooking Time: 0 minutes

Servings: 4

Ingredients:

- 3 cups pineapple, cored, sliced, and chunks
- 10–12 mint leaves, or to taste
- 2 tbsp. sugar, or to taste (optional)
- 1 ½ cup water
- 1 cup ice cubes

Directions:

1. Set all the ingredients into your blender, and pulse.
2. Set a fine-mesh strainer in a bowl. Before transferring your juice into the strainer.
3. Gently, press the pulp to extract all possible liquid, then discard it.
4. Serve over ice. Enjoy!

Nutrition:

- Calories: 78 kcal
- Fat: 1 g
- Carbs: 22 g
- Fiber: 2 g
- Protein: 1 g

9. Celery Apple Juice

Preparation Time: 5 minutes

Cooking Time: 0 minutes

Servings: 2

Ingredients:

- 12 celery stalks, peeled and chopped
- 3 Apple, peeled, cored, seeded, and sliced
- 1-inch ginger root, peeled and chopped
- 1/4 lemon juice
- 2 cups water

Directions:

1. Set all the ingredients into your blender, and pulse.

2. Set a fine-mesh strainer in a bowl. Before transferring your juice into the strainer.
3. Gently, press the pulp to extract all possible liquid, then discard it.
4. Serve over ice. Enjoy!

Nutrition:

- Calories: 119 kcal
- Fat: 1 g
- Carbs: 29 g
- Fiber: 7 g
- Protein: 2 g

10. Homemade Banana Apple Juice

Preparation Time: 10 minutes

Cooking Time: 0 minutes

Servings: 2

Ingredients:

- 2 bananas, peeled and sliced
- 1/2 apple, peeled, cored, and chopped
- 1 tbsp. honey
- 1 ½ cup water

Directions:

1. Set all the ingredients into your blender, and pulse.
2. Set a fine-mesh strainer in a bowl. Before transferring your juice into the strainer.
3. Gently, press the pulp to extract all possible liquid, then discard it.
4. Serve over ice. Enjoy!

Nutrition:

- Calories: 132 kcal
- Fat: 2 g
- Carbs: 27 g
- Fiber: 3 g
- Protein: 4 g

11. Sweet Detox Juice

Preparation Time: 10 minutes

Cooking Time: 0 minutes

Servings: 2

Ingredients:

- 2 cups baby spinach, chopped
- 1 handful parsley, chopped
- 1 green apple, peeled, cored, seeded, and sliced
- 1 large English cucumber, seeded and chopped
- 1-inch ginger, peeled
- 1 lemon, juiced

Directions:

1. Set all the ingredients into your blender, and pulse.
2. Set a fine-mesh strainer in a bowl. Before transferring your juice into the strainer.
3. Gently, press the pulp to extract all possible liquid, then discard it.
4. Serve over ice. Enjoy!

Nutrition:

- Calories: 209 kcal
- Fat: 2 g
- Carbs: 48 g
- Fiber: 17 g
- Protein: 12 g

12. Pineapple Ginger Juice

Preparation Time: 35 minutes

Cooking Time: 0 minutes

Servings: 7 cups

Ingredients:

- 10 cups pineapple, chopped
- 6 cups water
- 3 Fuji apples, chopped
- 4-inch ginger root, peeled and chopped
- 1/4 cup lemon juice
- 1/4 cup sugar

Directions:

1. Set all the ingredients into your blender, and pulse.
2. Set a fine-mesh strainer in a bowl. Before transferring your juice into the strainer.
3. Gently, press the pulp to extract all possible liquid, then discard it.
4. Serve over ice. Enjoy!

Nutrition:

- Calories: 71 kcal
- Fat: 1 g
- Carbs: 20 g
- Fiber: 3 g
- Protein: 1 g

13. Carrot Orange Juice

Preparation Time: 15 minutes

Cooking Time: 0 minutes

Servings: 2

Ingredients:

- 1 medium yellow tomato, cut into wedges
- 1 orange, peeled and quartered
- 1 apple, peeled, cored, and chopped
- 4 jumbo carrots, peeled and chopped
- 2 cups water

Directions:

1. Set all the ingredients into your blender, and pulse.
2. Set a fine-mesh strainer in a bowl. Before transferring your juice into the strainer.
3. Gently, press the pulp to extract all possible liquid, then discard it.
4. Serve over ice. Enjoy!

Nutrition:

- Calories: 111 kcal
- Fat: 1 g
- Carbs: 24 g
- Fiber: 1 g
- Protein: 2 g

14. Strawberry Apple Juice

Preparation Time: 5 minutes

Cooking Time: 0 minutes

Servings: 8–10 ounces

Ingredients:

- 2 cups strawberries (tops removed)
- 1 red apple, peeled, seeded, cored, and chopped
- 1 tbsp. chia seeds
- 1 cup water

Directions:

1. Set all the ingredients into your blender, and pulse.
2. Set a fine-mesh strainer in a bowl. Before transferring your juice into the strainer.
3. Gently, press the pulp to extract all possible liquid, then discard it.
4. Add in your chia seeds, then leave to sit for at least 5 minutes.
5. Serve over ice. Enjoy!

Nutrition:

- Calories: 245 kcal
- Fat: 5 g
- Carbs: 52 g
- Fiber: 7 g
- Protein: 4 g

15. Autumn Energizer Juice

Preparation Time: 10 minutes

Cooking Time: 0 minutes

Servings: 2

Ingredients:

- 2 pears, peeled, seeded, and chopped
- 2 Ambrosia apples, peeled, cored, and chopped

- 2 Granny Smith apples, peeled, cored, chopped
- 2 mandarins, juiced
- 2 cups sweet potato, peeled and chopped
- 1-pint cape gooseberries
- 2 inches ginger root, peeled

Directions:

1. Set all the ingredients into your blender, and pulse.
2. Set a fine-mesh strainer in a bowl. Before transferring your juice into the strainer.
3. Gently, press the pulp to extract all possible liquid, then discard it.
4. Serve over ice. Enjoy!

Nutrition:

- Calories: 170 kcal
- Fat: 3 g
- Carbs: 33 g
- Fiber: 9 g
- Protein: 4 g

16. Asian Inspired Wonton Broth

Preparation Time: 5 minutes

Cooking Time: 15 minutes

Servings: 2

Ingredients:

- 1 chicken thigh, skin on
- 1 carrot, coarsely chopped
- 1 celery stalk, coarsely chopped
- 1 small onion, quartered
- 3 dime-sized ginger pieces
- 2 tbsp. kosher salt
- 1/4 tsp. turmeric
- 1/8 tsp. MSG (don't leave it out)
- 5 white peppercorns (can be substituted with black)
- 1-liter water

Directions:

1. Transfer all the ingredients to your stockpot. Top with enough water to cover then allow to slowly come to a boil on high heat.
2. Switch to low heat and simmer for at least 15 minutes.
3. Set and pour the mixture through a fine-mesh strainer into a large bowl.
4. Taste and season with salt.
5. Serve hot.

Nutrition:

- Calories: 181 kcal
- Fat: 7 g
- Carbs: 14 g
- Fiber: 1 g
- Protein: 14 g

17. Mushroom, Cauliflower and Cabbage Broth

Preparation Time: 10 minutes

Cooking Time: 15 minutes

Servings: 2

Ingredients:

- 1 large yellow onion
- 1 cup celery stalks, chopped
- 2 carrots, diced or cubed
- 10 French beans
- 1/2 cabbage, diced
- 1–2 stalks celery leaves
- 1 ½ cup mushrooms, sliced
- 8 florets cauliflower
- 1 tsp. garlic, chopped
- 1 tsp. ginger, chopped
- 1 tbsp. oil
- 1 scallion stalk
- 1/2 tsp. pepper, crushed

Directions:

1. Transfer all the ingredients to your stockpot. Top with enough water to cover, then allow to slowly come to a boil on high heat.

2. Switch to low heat and simmer for 15 minutes.
3. Set and pour the mixture through a fine-mesh strainer into a large bowl. Mash the vegetables well to extract all their juices.
4. Taste and season with salt. Enjoy.

Nutrition:

- Calories: 141 kcal
- Fat: 5 g
- Carbs: 22 g
- Fiber: 7 g
- Protein: 5 g

18. Indian Inspired Vegetable Stock

Preparation Time: 10 minutes

Cooking Time: 11 minutes

Servings: 3

Ingredients:

- 3/4 cup onions, roughly chopped
- 3/4 cup carrot, roughly chopped
- 3/4 cup tomatoes, roughly chopped
- 3/4 cup potatoes, roughly chopped
- 1 tsp. turmeric
- Salt to taste

Directions:

1. Transfer all the ingredients to your stockpot. Top with enough water to cover, then allow to slowly come to a boil on high heat.
2. Switch to low heat and simmer for 11 minutes.
3. Set and pour the mixture through a fine-mesh strainer into a large bowl. Taste and season with salt.
4. Serve hot. Enjoy!

Nutrition:

- Calories: 103 kcal
- Fat: 0.2 mg
- Carbs: 23.3 g
- Fiber: 3.1 g
- Protein: 2.2 g

19. Beef Bone Broth

Preparation Time: 10 minutes

Cooking Time: 15 minutes

Servings: 8

Ingredients:

- 2 pounds beef bones
- 1 onion, chopped in quarters
- 2 celery stalks, chopped in half
- 2 carrots, chopped in half
- 3 whole garlic cloves
- 2 bay leaves
- 1 tbsp. salt
- Filtered water (enough to cover bones)

Directions:

1. Transfer the bones and vegetables to your stockpot. Top with enough water to cover, then allow to slowly come to a boil on high heat.
2. Switch to low heat and simmer for at least 15 minutes.
3. Set and pour the mixture through a fine-mesh strainer into a large bowl. Taste and season with salt.
4. Serve hot.

Nutrition:

- Calories: 69 kcal
- Fat: 4 g
- Carbs: 1 g
- Fiber: 0.1 g
- Protein: 6 g

20. Ginger, Mushroom and Cauliflower Broth

Preparation Time: 10 minutes

Cooking Time: 15 minutes

Servings: 3

Ingredients:

- 1 large yellow onion
- 1 cup celery stalks, chopped

- 2 carrots, diced or cubed
- 10 French beans
- 1 ginger root, peeled, diced, or grated
- 1–2 stalks celery leaves or coriander leaves
- 1 ½ cup mushrooms, sliced
- 8 florets cauliflower
- 1 tsp. garlic, chopped
- 1 tbsp. oil
- 1 stalk spring onion greens or scallions
- 1/2 tsp. crushed pepper or ground pepper

Directions:

1. Transfer all the ingredients to your stockpot. Top with enough water to cover, then allow to slowly come to a boil on high heat.
2. Switch to low heat and simmer for at least 15 minutes.
3. Set and pour the mixture through a fine-mesh strainer into a large bowl. Taste and season with salt.
4. Serve hot. Enjoy!

Nutrition:

- Calories: 141 kcal
- Fat: 5 g
- Carbs: 22 g
- Fiber: 7 g
- Protein: 5 g

21. Fish Broth

Preparation Time: 15 minutes

Cooking Time: 15 minutes

Servings: 3

Ingredients:

- 1 large onion, chopped
- 1 large carrot chopped
- 1 fennel bulb and fronds, chopped (optional)
- 3 celery stalks, chopped
- Salt
- 2–5 pounds fish bones and heads
- 1 handful dried mushrooms (optional)
- 2–4 bay leaves
- 1-star anise pod (optional)
- 1–2 tsp. thyme, dried or fresh
- 3–4 pieces dried kombu kelp (optional)

Directions:

1. Transfer the bones and vegetables to your stockpot. Top with enough water to cover, then allow to slowly come to a boil on high heat.
2. Set to low heat and simmer for 45 minutes.
3. Set and pour the mixture through a fine-mesh strainer into a large bowl. Taste and season with salt.
4. Serve hot. Enjoy!

Nutrition:

- Calories: 29 kcal
- Fat: 1 g
- Carbs: 2 g
- Fiber: 1 g
- Protein: 1 g

22. Clear Pumpkin Broth

Preparation Time: 15 minutes

Cooking Time: 15 minutes

Servings: 6

Ingredients:

- 6 cups water
- 2 tbsp. ginger, minced
- 2 cups potatoes, peeled and diced
- 3 cups kabocha, peeled and diced
- 1 carrot, peeled and diced
- 1 onion, diced
- 1/2 cup scallions, chopped

Directions:

1. Transfer the bones and vegetables to your stockpot. Top with enough water to cover, then allow to slowly come to a boil on high heat.

2. Switch to low heat and simmer for at least 15 minutes.
3. Set and pour the mixture through a fine-mesh strainer into a large bowl. Taste and season with salt.
4. Serve hot. Enjoy!

Nutrition:

- Calories: 216 kcal
- Fat: 1 g
- Carbs: 37 g
- Fiber: 4 g
- Protein: 8 g

23. Healthier Apple Juice

Preparation Time: 5 minutes

Cooking Time: 0 minutes

Servings: 2

Ingredients:

- 8 medium apples, cored and quartered

Directions:

1. Add the apples into a juicer and extract the juice according to the manufacturer's method.
2. Through a cheesecloth-lined sieve, strain the juice and transfer it into 2 glasses.
3. Serve immediately.

Nutrition:

- Calories: 164 kcal
- Carbs: 123.6 g
- Protein: 2.4 g
- Fat: 1.6 g
- Sugar: 90 g
- Sodium: 123 mg
- Fiber: 21.6 g

24. Citrus Apple Juice

Preparation Time: 5 minutes

Cooking Time: 0 minutes

Servings: 2

Ingredients:

- 5 large apples, cored and chopped
- 1 small lemon
- 1 cup fresh orange juice

Directions:

1. Attach all the ingredients in a blender and pulse until well combined.
2. Through a cheesecloth-lined sieve, strain the juice and transfer it into 2 glasses.
3. Serve immediately.

Nutrition:

- Calories: 148 kcal
- Carbs: 90.6 g
- Protein: 2.4 g
- Fat: 1.3 g
- Sugar: 68.6g
- Sodium: 6 mg
- Fiber: 14 g

25. Richly Fruity Juice

Preparation Time: 15 minutes

Cooking Time: 10 minutes

Servings: 2

Ingredients:

- 5 large green apples, cored and sliced
- 2 cups seedless white grapes
- 2 tsp. fresh lime juice

Directions:

1. Set all ingredients into a juicer and extract the juice according to the manufacturer's method.
2. Through a cheesecloth-lined sieve, strain the juice and transfer it into 2 glasses.
3. Serve immediately.

Nutrition:

- Calories: 152 kcal
- Carbs: 92.8 g
- Protein: 2.1 g
- Fat: 1.3 g
- Sugar: 73 g
- Sodium: 7 mg

- Fiber: 14.3 g

26. Delish Grape Juice

Preparation Time: 15 minutes

Cooking Time: 0 minutes

Servings: 3

Ingredients:

- 2 cups white seedless grapes
- 1 ½ cup filtered water
- 6–8 ice cubes

Directions:

1. Attach all the ingredients in a blender and pulse until well combined.
2. Through a cheesecloth-lined sieve, strain the juice and transfer it into 3 glasses.
3. Serve immediately.

Nutrition:

- Calories: 41 kcal
- Carbs: 10.5 g
- Protein: 0.4 g
- Fat: 0.2 g
- Sugar: 10 g
- Sodium: 1 mg
- Fiber: 10 g

27. Lemony Grape Juice

Preparation Time: 15 minutes

Cooking Time: 0 minutes

Servings: 3

Ingredients:

- 4 cups seedless white grapes
- 2 tbsp. fresh lemon juice

Directions:

1. Attach all the ingredients in a blender and pulse until well combined.
2. Through a cheesecloth-lined sieve, strain the juice and transfer it into 3 glasses.
3. Serve immediately.

Nutrition:

- Calories: 85 kcal
- Carbs: 21.3 g
- Protein: 0.9 g
- Fat: 0.5 g
- Sugar: 20.1 g
- Sodium: 4 mg
- Fiber: 1.1 g

28. Holiday Special Juice

Preparation Time: 15 minutes

Cooking Time: 0 minutes

Servings: 4

Ingredients:

- 4 cups fresh cranberries
- 1 tbsp. fresh lemon juice
- 2 cups filtered water
- 1 tsp. raw honey

Directions:

1. Attach all the ingredients in a blender and pulse until well combined.
2. Through a cheesecloth-lined sieve, strain the juice and transfer it into 4 glasses.
3. Serve immediately.

Nutrition:

- Calories: 66 kcal
- Carbs: 11.5 g
- Protein: 0 g
- Fat: 0 g
- Sugar: 5.5 g
- Sodium: 1 mg
- Fiber: 4 g

29. Vitamin C Rich Juice

Preparation Time: 15 minutes

Cooking Time: 0 minutes

Servings: 2

Ingredients:

- 8 oranges, peeled and sectioned

Directions:

1. Add the orange sections into a juicer and extract the juice according to the manufacturer's method.
2. Through a cheesecloth-lined sieve, strain the juice and transfer it into 2 glasses.
3. Serve immediately.

Nutrition:

- Calories: 146 kcal
- Carbs: 86.5 g
- Protein: 6.9 g
- Fat: 0.9 g
- Sugar: 68.8 g
- Sodium: 0 mg
- Fiber: 17.7 g

30. Incredible Fresh Juice

Preparation Time: 15 minutes

Cooking Time: 0 minutes

Servings: 4

Ingredients:

- 2 pounds carrots, trimmed and scrubbed
- 6 small oranges, peeled and sectioned

Directions:

1. Add the carrots and orange sections into a juicer and extract the juice according to the manufacturer's method.
2. Through a cheesecloth-lined sieve, strain the juice and transfer it into 4 glasses.
3. Serve immediately.

Nutrition:

- Calories: 183 kcal
- Carbs: 44.9 g
- Protein: 3.7 g
- Fat: 0.2 g
- Sugar: 29.1 g
- Sodium: 156 mg
- Fiber: 10.2 g

31. Favorite Summer Lemonade

Preparation Time: 15 minutes

Cooking Time: 0 minutes

Servings: 8

Ingredients:

- 8 cups filtered water
- 1/2 cup fresh lemon juice
- 1/4 tsp. pure stevia extract
- Ice cubes, as required

Directions:

1. In a pitcher, place the water, lemon juice, and stevia. Mix well.
2. Through a cheesecloth-lined sieve, strain the lemonade in another pitcher.
3. Refrigerate for 30–40 minutes.
4. Set ice cubes in serving glasses and fill with lemonade.
5. Serve chilled.

Nutrition:

- Calories: 4 kcal
- Carbs: 0.3 g
- Protein: 0.1 g
- Fat: 0.1 g
- Sugar: 0.3 g
- Sodium: 3 mg
- Fiber: 0.1 g

32. Ultimate Fruity Punch

Preparation Time: 15 minutes

Cooking Time: 0 minutes

Servings: 12

Ingredients:

- 3 cups fresh pineapple juice
- 2 cups fresh orange juice
- 1 cup fresh ruby red grapefruit juice
- 1/4 cup fresh lime juice

- 2 cups seedless watermelon, cut into bite-sized chunks
- 2 cups fresh pineapple, cut into bite-sized chunks
- 2 oranges, peeled and cut into wedges
- 2 limes, quartered
- 1 lemon, sliced
- 2 (12 ounces) cans diet lemon-lime soda
- Crushed ice, as required

Directions:

1. In a large pitcher, add all ingredients except for soda cans and ice. Stir to combine.
2. Set aside for 30 minutes.
3. Through a cheesecloth-lined sieve, strain the punch into another large pitcher.
4. Set the glasses with ice and top with punch about 3/4 of the mixture.
5. Add a splash of the soda and serve.

Nutrition:

- Calories: 95 kcal
- Carbs: 23.4 g
- Protein: 1.3 g
- Fat: 0.3 g
- Sugar: 18.3 g
- Sodium: 152 mg
- Fiber: 1.8 g

33. Thirst Quencher Sports Drink

Preparation Time: 15 minutes

Cooking Time: 0 minutes

Servings: 8

Ingredients:

- 7 cups spring water
- 1 cup fresh apple juice
- 2–3 tsp. fresh lime juice
- 2 tbsp. honey
- 1/4 tsp. sea salt

Directions:

1. In a large pitcher, add all ingredients and stir to combine.
2. Through a cheesecloth-lined sieve, strain the punch into another large pitcher.
3. Refrigerate to chill before serving.

Nutrition:

- Calories: 30 kcal
- Carbs: 7.8 g
- Protein: 0.1 g
- Fat: 0 g
- Sugar: 7.3 g
- Sodium: 60 mg
- Fiber: 0.1 g

34. Refreshing Sports Drink

Preparation Time: 15 minutes

Cooking Time: 0 minutes

Servings: 9

Ingredients:

- 8 cups fresh cold water, divided
- 3/4 cup fresh orange juice
- 1/4 cup fresh lemon juice
- 1/4 cup fresh limes juice
- 3 tbsp. honey
- 1/2 tsp. salt

Directions:

1. In a large pitcher, add all ingredients and stir to combine.
2. Through a cheesecloth-lined sieve, strain the punch into another large pitcher.
3. Refrigerate to chill before serving.

Nutrition:

- Calories: 33 kcal
- Carbs: 8.1 g
- Protein: 0.2 g
- Fat: 0.1 g
- Sugar: 7.6 g
- Sodium: 130 mg

- Fiber: 0.1 g

35. Perfect Sunny Day Tea

Preparation Time: 15 minutes
Cooking Time: 3 minutes
Servings: 6
Ingredients:

- 5 cups filtered water
- 5 green tea bags
- 1/4 cup fresh lemon juice, strained
- 1/4 cup fresh lime juice, strained
- 1/4 cup honey
- Ice cubes, as required

Directions:

1. In a medium pan, add 2 cups of water and bring to a boil.
2. Set in the tea bags and turn off the heat.
3. Immediately, cover the pan and steep for 3–4 minutes.
4. With a large spoon, gently press the tea bags against the pan to extract the tea completely.
5. Detach the tea bags from the pan and discard them.
6. Set honey and stir until dissolved.
7. In a large pitcher, place the tea, lemon, and lime juice and stir to combine.
8. Add the remaining cold water and stir to combine.
9. Refrigerate to chill before serving.
10. Attach ice cubes in serving glasses and fill with tea.
11. Serve chilled.

Nutrition:

- Calories: 46 kcal
- Carbs: 12 g
- Protein: 0.1 g
- Fat: 0.1 g
- Sugar: 11.8 g
- Sodium: 3 mg
- Fiber: 0.1 g

36. Nutritious Green Tea

Preparation Time: 15 minutes
Cooking Time: 4 minutes
Servings: 4
Ingredients:

- 4 cups filtered water
- 4 orange peel strips
- 4 lemon peel strips
- 4 green tea bags
- 2 tsp. honey

Directions:

1. In a medium pan, add the water, orange, and lemon peel strips over medium-high heat and bring to a boil.
2. Set the heat to low and stir, uncovered, for about 10 minutes.
3. With a slotted spoon, remove the orange and lemon peel strips and discard them.
4. Attach in the tea bags and turn off the heat.
5. Immediately, cover the pan and steep for 3 minutes.
6. With a large spoon, gently press the tea bags against the pan to extract the tea completely.
7. Detach the tea bags from the pan and discard them.
8. Add honey and stir until dissolved.
9. Strain the tea in mugs and serve immediately.

Nutrition:

- Calories: 11 kcal
- Carbs: 3 g
- Protein: 0 g
- Fat: 0 g
- Sugar: 2.9 g
- Sodium: 0 mg
- Fiber: 0.1 g

37. Simple Black Tea

Preparation Time: 10 minutes

Cooking Time: 3 minutes

Servings: 2

Ingredients:

- 2 cups filtered water
- 1/2 tsp. black tea leaves
- 1 tsp. honey

Directions:

1. In a pan, add the water and bring to a boil.
2. Stir in the tea leaves and turn off the heat.
3. Immediately, cover the pan and steep for 3 minutes.
4. Add honey and stir until dissolved.
5. Strain the tea in mugs and serve immediately.

Nutrition:

- Calories: 11 kcal
- Carbs: 2.9 g
- Protein: 0 g
- Fat: 0 g
- Sugar: 2.9 g
- Sodium: 123 mg
- Fiber: 0 g

38. Lemony Black Tea

Preparation Time: 10 minutes

Cooking Time: 3 minutes

Servings: 6

Ingredients:

- 1 tbsp. black tea leaves
- 1 lemon, sliced thinly
- 1 cinnamon stick
- 6 cups boiling water

Directions:

1. In a large teapot, place the tea leaves, lemon slices, and cinnamon stick.
2. Pour hot water over the ingredients and immediately cover the teapot.
3. Set aside for about 5 minutes to steep.
4. Strain the tea in mugs and serve immediately.

Nutrition:

- Calories: 1
- Carbs: 0.2 g
- Protein: 0 g
- Fat: 0 g
- Sugar: 0.1 g
- Sodium: 0 mg
- Fiber: 0.1 g

39. Metabolism Booster Coffee

Preparation Time: 5 minutes

Cooking Time: 4 minutes

Servings: 1

Ingredients:

- 1/4 tsp. coffee powder
- 1 ¼ cup filtered water
- 1 tsp. fresh lemon juice
- 1 tsp. honey

Directions:

1. In a small pan, attach the water and coffee powder. Bring it to boil.
2. Cook for about 1 minute.
3. Detach from the heat and pour into a serving mug.
4. Add the honey and lemon juice, then stir until dissolved
5. Serve hot.

Nutrition:

- Calories: 23 kcal
- Carbs: 6 g
- Protein: 0.1 g
- Fat: 0 g
- Sugar: 5.9 g
- Sodium: 1 mg
- Fiber: 0 g

40. Best Homemade Broth

Preparation Time: 15 minutes

Cooking Time: 15 minutes

Servings: 8

Ingredients:

- 1 (3 pounds) chicken, cut into pieces
- 5 medium carrots
- 4 celery stalks with leaves
- 6 fresh thyme sprigs
- 6 fresh parsley sprigs
- Salt to taste
- 9 cups cold water

Directions:

1. In a large pan, attach all the ingredients over medium-high heat and bring to a boil.
2. Set the heat to medium-low and stir, covered for about 15 minutes, occasionally skimming the foam from the surface.
3. Through a fine-mesh sieve, strain the broth into a large bowl.
4. Serve hot.

Nutrition:

- Calories: 275 kcal
- Carbs: 4.3 g
- Protein: 49.7 g
- Fat: 5.2 g
- Sugar: 2 g
- Sodium: 160 mg
- Fiber: 1.2 g

41. Clean Testing Broth

Preparation Time: 5 hours 50 minutes

Cooking Time: 15 minutes

Servings: 10

Ingredients:

- 4 pounds chicken bones
- Salt to taste
- 10 cups filtered water
- 2 tbsp. apple cider vinegar
- 1 lemon, quartered
- 3 bay leaves
- 3 tsp. ground turmeric
- 2 tbsp. peppercorns

Directions:

1. Preheat the oven to 400ºF.
2. Arrange the bones onto a large baking sheet and sprinkle with salt.
3. Roast for about 45 minutes.
4. Detach from the oven and transfer the bones into a large pan.
5. Add the remaining ingredients and stir to combine.
6. Put the pan over medium-high heat and bring to a boil.
7. Set the heat to low and stir, covered for about 4–5 hours, occasionally skimming the foam from the surface.
8. Through a fine-mesh sieve, strain the broth into a large bowl.
9. Serve hot.

Nutrition:

- Calories: 140 kcal
- Carbs: 0.6 g
- Protein: 25 g
- Fat: 2.6 g
- Sugar: 0.1 g
- Sodium: 73 mg
- Fiber: 0.1 g

42. Healing Broth

Preparation Time: 10 hours 25 minutes

Cooking Time: 15 minutes

Servings: 12

Ingredients:

- 3 tbsp. extra-virgin olive oil
- 2 ½ pounds chicken bones
- 4 celery stalks, chopped roughly
- 3 large carrots, peeled and chopped roughly
- 1 bay leaf
- 1 tbsp. black peppercorns
- 2 whole cloves

- 1 tbsp. apple cider vinegar
- Warm water, as required

Directions:

1. In a Dutch oven, heat the oil over medium-high heat and sear the bones for about 3–5 minutes or until browned.
2. With a slotted spoon, transfer the bones into a bowl.
3. In the same pan, add the celery stalks and carrots. Cook for about 15 minutes, stirring occasionally.
4. Add browned bones, bay leaf, black peppercorns, cloves, and vinegar. Stir to combine.
5. Add enough warm water to cover the bones mixture completely and bring to a gentle boil.
6. Set the heat to low and stir, covered for about 8–10 hours, occasionally skimming the foam from the surface.
7. Through a fine-mesh sieve, strain the broth into a large bowl.
8. Serve hot.

Nutrition:

- Calories: 67 kcal
- Carbs: 2 g
- Protein: 5.7 g
- Fat: 4.1 g
- Sugar: 1 g
- Sodium: 29 mg
- Fiber: 0.5 g

43. Veggie Lover's Broth

Preparation Time: 2 hours 5 minutes

Cooking Time: 15 minutes

Servings: 10

Ingredients:

- 4 carrots, peeled and chopped roughly
- 4 celery stalks, chopped roughly
- 3 parsnips, peeled and chopped roughly
- 2 large potatoes, peeled and chopped roughly
- 1 medium beet, trimmed and chopped roughly
- 1 large bunch fresh parsley
- 1 (1 inch) piece fresh ginger, sliced
- Filtered water, as required

Directions:

1. In a pan, add all the ingredients over medium-high heat.
2. Add enough water to cover the veggie mixture and bring to a boil.
3. Set the heat to low and simmer, covered for about 2–3 hours.
4. Through a fine-mesh sieve, strain the broth into a large bowl.
5. Serve hot.

Nutrition:

- Calories: 82 kcal
- Carbs: 19 g
- Protein: 1.9 g
- Fat: 0.2 g
- Sugar: 3.9 g
- Sodium: 37 mg
- Fiber: 3.7 g

44. Brain Healthy Broth

Preparation Time: 12 hours 5 minutes

Cooking Time: 10 minutes

Servings: 6

Ingredients:

- 12 cups filtered water
- 2 pounds non-oily fish heads and bones
- 1/4 cup apple cider vinegar
- Sea salt to taste

Directions:

1. In a large pan, attach all the ingredients over medium-high heat.
2. Add enough water to cover the veggie mixture and bring to a boil.
3. Set the heat to low and simmer, covered for about 15 minutes, occasionally skimming the foam from the surface.

4. Through a fine-mesh sieve, strain the broth into a large bowl.
5. Serve hot.

Nutrition:

- Calories: 75 kcal
- Carbs: 0.1 g
- Protein: 13.4 g
- Fat: 1.7 g
- Sugar: 0 g
- Sodium: 253 mg
- Fiber: 0 g

45. Minerals Rich Broth

Preparation Time: 15 minutes

Cooking Time: 15 minutes

Servings: 8

Ingredients:

- 5–7 pounds non-oily fish carcasses and heads
- 2 tbsp. olive oil
- 3 carrots, scrubbed and chopped roughly
- 2 celery stalks, chopped roughly

Directions:

1. In a pan, heat the oil over medium-low heat and cook the carrots and celery for about 20 minutes, stirring occasionally.
2. Add the fish bones and enough water to cover by 1-inch and stir to combine.
3. Set the heat to medium-high and bring to a boil.
4. Set the heat to low, cover, and cook for about 1–2 hours, occasionally skimming the foam from the surface.
5. Through a fine-mesh sieve, strain the broth into a large bowl.
6. Serve hot.

Nutrition:

- Calories: 113 kcal
- Carbs: 2.5 g
- Protein: 13.7 g
- Fat: 5.2 g
- Sugar: 1.2 g
- Sodium: 234 mg
- Fiber: 0.7 g

46. Holiday Favorite Gelatin

Preparation Time: 15 minutes

Cooking Time: 15 minutes

Servings: 6

Ingredients:

- 1 tbsp. grass-fed gelatin powder
- 1 ¾ cup fresh apple juice, warmed
- 1/4 cup boiling water
- 1–2 drops fresh lemon juice

Directions:

1. In a medium bowl, pour in the tbsp. of gelatin powder.
2. Add just enough warm apple juice to cover the gelatin and stir well.
3. Set aside for about 2–3 minutes or until it forms a thick syrup.
4. Add 1/4 cup of the boiling water and stir until gelatin is dissolved completely.
5. Add the remaining juice and lemon juice then stir well.
6. Transfer the mixture into a parchment paper-lined baking dish and refrigerate for 2 hours or until the top is firm before serving.

Nutrition:

- Calories: 40 kcal
- Carbs: 8.2 g
- Protein: 1.9 g
- Fat: 0.1 g
- Sugar: 7 g
- Sodium: 5 mg
- Fiber: 0.2 g

47. Chicken Bone Broth

Preparation Time: 10 minutes

Cooking Time: 15 minutes

Servings: 8

Ingredients:

- 3–4 pounds bones (from 1 chicken)
- 4 cups water
- 2 large carrots, cut into chunks
- 2 large stalks celery
- 1 large onion
- 2 cups Fresh rosemary sprigs
- 3 fresh thyme sprigs
- 2 tbsp. apple cider vinegar
- 1 tsp. kosher salt

Directions:

1. Put all the ingredients in your pot and allow to sit for 10 minutes.
2. Pressure cook and adjust the time to 15 minutes.
3. Set the release naturally until the float valve drops and then unlock the lid.
4. Strain the broth and transfer it into a storage container. The broth can be refrigerated for 3–5 days or frozen for up to 6 months.

Nutrition:

- Calories: 140 kcal
- Carbs: 0.6 g
- Protein: 25 g
- Fat: 2.6 g
- Sugar: 0.1 g
- Sodium: 73 mg
- Fiber: 0.1 g

48. Homemade Beef Stock

Preparation Time: 10 minutes

Cooking Time: 15 minutes

Servings: 6

Ingredients:

- 2 pounds beef bones (preferably with marrow)
- 5 celery stalks, chopped
- 4 carrots, chopped
- 1 white or Spanish onion, chopped
- 2 garlic cloves, crushed
- 2 bay leaves
- 1 tsp. dried thyme
- 1 tsp. dried sage
- 1 tsp. black peppercorns
- Salt

Directions:

1. Preheat the oven to 425ºF.
2. On a baking sheet, spread out the beef bones, celery, carrots, onion, garlic, and bay leaves. Sprinkle the thyme, sage, and peppercorns over the top.
3. Roast until the vegetables and bones have a rich brown color.
4. Transfer the roasted bones and vegetables to a large stockpot. Cover with water and slowly bring to a boil over high heat.
5. Set the heat to medium-low for at least 15 minutes.
6. Pour the mixture through a fine-mesh strainer into a large bowl.
7. Taste and season with salt. Serve hot.

Nutrition:

- Calories: 37 kcal
- Fat: 1 g
- Carbs: 3 g
- Fiber: 0 g
- Protein: 4 g
- Sodium: 58 mg

49. Three-Ingredient Sugar-Free Gelatin

Preparation Time: 5 minutes

Cooking Time: 0 minutes

Servings: 6–8

Ingredients:

- 1/4 cup room temperature water
- 1/4 cup hot water
- 1 tbsp. gelatin
- 1 cup orange juice, unsweetened

Directions:

1. Combine your gelatin and room temperature water, stirring until fully dissolved.
2. Stir in hot water, then leave to rest for about 2 minutes.
3. Add in the juice and stir until combined.
4. Transfer to serving size containers, then place on a tray in the refrigerator to set for about 4 hours.
5. Enjoy!

Nutrition:

- Calories: 17 kcal
- Fat: 0 g
- Carbs: 4 g
- Fiber: 0 g
- Protein: 0 g

50. Cranberry-Kombucha Jell-O

Preparation Time: 5 minutes

Cooking Time: 0 minutes

Servings: 6

Ingredients:

- 1/4 cup room temperature water
- 1/4 cup hot water
- 1 tbsp. gelatin
- 1 cup cranberry kombucha, unsweetened

Directions:

1. Combine your gelatin and room temperature water, stirring until fully dissolved.
2. Stir in hot water, then leave to rest for about 2 minutes.
3. Add in the kombucha and stir until combined.
4. Transfer to serving size containers, then place on a tray in the refrigerator to set for about 4 hours.
5. Enjoy!

Nutrition:

- Calories: 13
- Fat: 0 g
- Carbs: 1 g
- Fiber: 0 g
- Protein: 0 g

51. Strawberry Gummies

Preparation Time: 5 minutes

Cooking Time: 5 minutes

Servings: 20–40 mini gummies

Ingredients:

- 1 cup strawberries, hulled and chopped
- 3/4 cup water
- 2 tbsp. gelatin

Directions:

1. Bring your water and berries to a boil on high heat. Detach from the heat as soon as the mixture begins to boil.
2. Transfer to the blender and pulse. Add in your gelatin, then blend once more.
3. Pour the mixture into a gummy silicone mold.
4. Place on a tray in the refrigerator to set for about 4 hours.
5. Enjoy!

Nutrition:

- Calories: 3 kcal
- Fat: 0 g
- Carbs: 0 g
- Fiber: 0 g
- Protein: 0 g

52. Fruity Jell-O Stars

Preparation Time: 15 minutes

Cooking Time: 5 minutes

Servings: 4

Ingredients:

- 1 tbsp. gelatin, powdered
- 3/4 cup boiling water
- 3 ½ cups fruit
- 1 tbsp. honey
- 1 tsp. lemon juice

Directions:

1. Attach all your ingredients into a blender and pulse.
2. Add in the gelatin, then blend once more.
3. Pour the mixture into a gummy silicone mold.
4. Place on a tray in the refrigerator to set for about 4 hours.
5. Enjoy!

Nutrition:

- Calories: 2 kcal
- Fat: 14 g
- Carbs: 0 g
- Fiber: 1 g
- Protein: 0 g

53. Sugar-Free Cinnamon Jelly

Preparation Time: 5 minutes

Cooking Time: 0 minutes

Servings: 2

Ingredients:

- 1 cup hot cinnamon tea
- 1 cup room temperature water
- 2 tsp. gelatin
- 1/3 cup sweetener

Directions:

1. Combine your gelatin and room temperature water, stirring until fully dissolved.
2. Stir in hot tea, then leave to rest for about 2 minutes.
3. Add in the sweetener and stir until combined.
4. Transfer to serving size containers, then place on a tray in the refrigerator to set for about 4 hours.
5. Enjoy!

Nutrition:

- Calories: 35 kcal
- Fat: 0 g
- Carbs: 17 g
- Fiber: 0 g
- Protein: 0 g

54. Homey Clear Chicken Broth

Preparation Time: 10 minutes

Cooking Time: 15 minutes

Servings: 6 cups

Ingredients:

- 2 pounds chicken neck
- 2 celery ribs with leaves, cut into chunks
- 2 medium carrots, cut into chunks
- 2 medium onions, quartered
- 2 bay leaves
- 2 quarts cold water
- Salt

Directions:

1. Transfer the bones and vegetables to your stockpot. Top with enough water to cover, then allow to slowly come to a boil on high heat.
2. Switch to low heat and simmer for at least 15 minutes.
3. Set and pour the mixture through a fine-mesh strainer into a large bowl.
4. Taste and season with salt.
5. Serve hot.

Nutrition:

- Calories: 245 kcal

- Fat: 14 g
- Carbs: 8 g
- Fiber: 2 g
- Protein: 21 g

55. Oxtail Bone Broth

Preparation Time: 15 minutes

Cooking Time: 15 minutes

Servings: 8 cups

Ingredients:

- 2 pounds Oxtail
- 1 Onion, chopped in quarters
- 2 celery stalks, chopped in half
- 2 carrots, chopped in half
- 3 whole garlic cloves
- 2 bay leaves
- 1 tbsp. salt
- Filtered water (enough to cover bones)

Directions:

1. Transfer the bones and vegetables to your stockpot. Top with enough water to cover, then allow to slowly come to a boil on high heat.
2. Switch to low heat and simmer for at least 15 minutes.
3. Set and pour the mixture through a fine-mesh strainer into a large bowl.
4. Taste and season with salt.
5. Serve hot.

Nutrition:

- Calories: 576 kcal
- Fat: 48 g
- Carbs: 48 g
- Fiber: 0 g
- Protein: 24 g

56. Chicken Bone Broth with Ginger and Lemon

Preparation Time: 10 minutes

Cooking Time: 15 minutes

Servings: 8

Ingredients:

- 3–4 pounds bones (from 1 chicken)
- 8 cups water
- 2 large carrots, cut into chunks
- 2 large stalks celery
- 1 large onion
- 3 fresh rosemary sprigs
- 3 fresh thyme sprigs
- 2 tbsp. apple cider vinegar
- 1 tsp. kosher salt
- 1 (1/2 inches) piece fresh ginger, sliced (peeling not necessary)
- 1 large lemon, cut into quarters

Directions:

1. Put all the ingredients in your pot and allow to sit for 10 minutes.
2. Pressure cook and adjust the time to 15 minutes.
3. Set the broth using a fine-mesh strainer and transfer it into a storage container.
4. Can be refrigerated for 5 days or frozen for 6 months.

Nutrition:

- Calories: 44 kcal
- Fat: 1 g
- Protein: 7 g
- Sodium: 312 mg
- Fiber: 0 g
- Carbs: 0 g
- Sugar: 0 g

57. Vegetable Stock

Preparation Time: 10 minutes

Cooking Time: 15 minutes

Servings: 8

Ingredients:

- 2 large carrots
- 1 large onion
- 2 large stalks celery
- 8 ounces white mushrooms
- 5 whole garlic cloves

- 2 cups parsley leaves
- 2 bay leaves
- 2 tsp. whole black peppercorns
- 2 tsp. kosher salt
- 10 cups water

Directions:

1. Place all the ingredients in your pot. Secure the lid.
2. Pressure cook and adjust the time to 15 minutes.
3. Set the broth using a fine-mesh strainer and transfer it into a storage container.

Nutrition:

- Calories: 9 kcal
- Fat: 0 g
- Protein: 0 g
- Sodium: 585 mg
- Fiber: 0 g
- Carbs: 2 g
- Sugar: 1 g

58. Chicken Vegetable Soup

Preparation Time: 23 minutes

Cooking Time: 15 minutes

Servings: 8

Ingredients:

- 2 tbsp. avocado oil
- 1 small yellow onion, peeled and chopped
- 2 large carrots, peeled and chopped
- 2 large stalks celery, ends removed and sliced
- 3 garlic cloves, minced
- 1 tsp. dried thyme
- 1 tsp. salt
- 8 cups chicken stock
- 3 boneless, skinless, frozen chicken breasts

Directions:

1. Heat the oil for 1 minute. Add the onion, carrots, and celery and saute for 8 minutes.
2. Add the garlic, thyme, and salt, then saute for another 30 seconds. Press the Cancel button.
3. Add the stock and frozen chicken breasts to the pot. Secure the lid.
4. Pressure cook and adjust the time to 6 minutes.
5. Allow cooling into bowls to serve.

Nutrition:

- Calories: 209 kcal
- Fat: 7 g
- Protein: 21 g
- Sodium: 687 mg
- Fiber: 1 g
- Carbs: 12 g
- Sugar: 5 g

59. Carrot Ginger Soup

Preparation Time: 20 minutes

Cooking Time: 15 minutes

Servings: 4

Ingredients:

- 1 tbsp. avocado oil
- 1 large yellow onion, peeled and chopped
- 1 pound carrots, peeled and chopped
- 1 tbsp. fresh ginger, peeled and minced
- 1 ½ tsp. salt
- 3 cups vegetable broth

Directions:

1. Add the oil to the inner pot, allowing it to heat for 1 minute.
2. Attach the onion, carrots, ginger, and salt, then saute for 5 minutes. Press the Cancel button.
3. Add the broth and secure the lid. Adjust the time to 10 minutes.
4. Allow the soup to cool a few minutes, and then transfer it to a large blender.

Merge on high until smooth and then serve.

Nutrition:

- Calories: 99 kcal
- Fat: 4 g
- Protein: 1 g
- Sodium: 1.348 mg
- Fiber: 4 g
- Carbs: 16 g
- Sugar: 7 g

60. Turkey Sweet Potato Hash

Preparation Time: 10 minutes

Cooking Time: 12 minutes

Servings: 4

Ingredients:

- 1 ½ tbsp. avocado oil
- 1 medium yellow onion, peeled and diced
- 2 garlic cloves, minced
- 1 medium sweet potato, cut into cubes (peeling not necessary)
- 1/2 pound lean ground turkey
- 1/2 tsp. salt
- 1 tsp. Italian seasoning blend

Directions:

1. Attach the oil and allow it to heat for 1 minute. Add the onion and cook until softened, about 5 minutes. Attach the garlic and cook for an additional 30 seconds.
2. Add the sweet potato, turkey, salt, and Italian seasoning and cook for another 5 minutes.

Nutrition:

- Calories: 172 kcal
- Fat: 9 g
- Protein: 12 g
- Sodium: 348 mg
- Fiber: 1 g
- Carbs: 10 g
- Sugar: 3 g

61. Chicken Tenders with Honey Mustard Sauce

Preparation Time: 5 minutes

Cooking Time: 10 minutes

Servings: 4

Ingredients:

- 1 pound chicken tenders
- 1 tbsp. fresh thyme leaves
- 1/2 tsp. salt
- 1/4 tsp. black pepper
- 1 tbsp. avocado oil
- 1 cup chicken stock
- 1/4 cup Dijon mustard
- 1/4 cup raw honey

Directions:

1. Dry the chicken tenders with a towel and then season them with thyme, salt, and pepper.
2. Attach the oil and let it heat for 2 minutes. Add the chicken tenders and seer them until brown on both sides, about 1 minute per side. Press the Cancel button.
3. Remove the chicken tenders and set them aside. Add the stock to the pot. Use a spoon to scrape up any small bits from the bottom of the pot.
4. Set the steam rack in the inner pot and place the chicken tenders directly on the rack.
5. While the chicken is cooking, prepare the sauce.
6. In a bowl, combine the Dijon mustard and honey, then stir to combine.
7. Serve the chicken tenders with the honey mustard sauce.

Nutrition:

- Calories: 223 kcal
- Fat: 5 g

- Protein: 22 g
- Sodium: 778 mg
- Fiber: 0 g
- Carbs: 19 g
- Sugar: 18 g

62. Chicken Breasts with Cabbage and Mushrooms

Preparation Time: 10 minutes

Cooking Time: 15 minutes

Servings: 4

Ingredients:

- 2 tbsp. avocado oil
- 1 pound sliced Baby Bella mushrooms
- 1 ½ tsp. salt, divided
- 2 garlic cloves, minced
- 8 cups chopped green cabbage
- 1 ½ tsp. dried thyme
- 1/2 cup chicken stock
- 1 ½ pound boneless, skinless chicken breasts

Directions:

1. Add the oil. Allow it to heat for 1 minute. Attach the mushrooms and 1/4 tsp. of salt. Saute until they have cooked down and released their liquid, about 10 minutes.
2. Add the garlic and saute for another 30 seconds. Press the Cancel button.
3. Attach the cabbage, 1/4 tsp. of salt, thyme, and the stock to the inner pot. Stir to combine.
4. Dry the chicken breasts and sprinkle both sides with the remaining salt. Place on top of the cabbage mixture.
5. Transfer to plates and spoon the juices on top.

Nutrition:

- Calories: 337 kcal
- Fat: 10 g
- Protein: 44 g
- Sodium: 1,023 mg
- Fiber: 4 g
- Carbs: 14 g
- Sugar: 2 g

63. Duck with Bok Choy

Preparation Time: 15 minutes

Cooking Time: 12 minutes

Servings: 6

Ingredients:

- 2 tbsp. coconut oil
- 1 onion, sliced thinly
- 2 tsp. fresh ginger, grated finely
- 2 minced garlic cloves
- 1 tbsp. fresh orange zest, grated finely
- 1/4 cup chicken broth
- 2/3 cup fresh orange juice
- 1 roasted duck, meat picked
- 3 pounds bok choy leaves
- 1 orange, peeled, seeded, and segmented

Directions:

1. In a sizable skillet, melt the coconut oil on medium heat. Attach the onion, saute for around 3 minutes. Add ginger and garlic, then saute for about 1–2 minutes.
2. Stir in the orange zest, broth, and orange juice.
3. Add the duck meat and cook for around 3 minutes.
4. Transfer the meat pieces to a plate. Add the bok choy and cook for about 3–4 minutes.
5. Divide the bok choy mixture into serving plates and top with duck meat.
6. Serve with the garnishing of orange segments.

Nutrition:

- Calories: 290 kcal
- Fat: 4 g
- Fiber: 6 g
- Carbs: 8 g

- Protein: 14 g

64. Beef with Mushroom and Broccoli

Preparation Time: 60 minutes

Cooking Time: 12 minutes

Servings: 4

Ingredients:

For Beef Marinade:

- 1 garlic clove, minced
- 1 piece fresh ginger, minced
- Salt and freshly ground black pepper
- 3 tbsp. white wine vinegar
- 3/4 cup beef broth
- 1 pound flank steak, trimmed and sliced into thin strips

For Vegetables:

- 2 tbsp. coconut oil
- 2 garlic cloves
- 3 cups broccoli rabe
- 4 ounces shiitake mushrooms
- 8 ounces cremini mushrooms

Directions:

For the marinade:

1. In a substantial bowl, mix all ingredients except the beef. Add it and coat with the marinade generously. Refrigerate to soak for around 1/4 hour.
2. In a substantial skillet, warm oil on medium-high heat.
3. Detach the beef from the bowl, reserving the marinade.

For the Vegetables:

1. Attach the beef and garlic and cook for about 3–4 minutes or till browned.
2. In the same skillet, add the reserved marinade, broccoli, and mushrooms. Cook for approximately 3–4 minutes.
3. Set in the beef and cook for about 3–4 minutes.

Nutrition:

- Calories: 200 kcal
- Carbs: 31 g
- Cholesterol: 93 mg
- Fat: 4 g
- Protein: 10 g
- Fiber: 2 g

65. Beef with Zucchini Noodles

Preparation Time: 15 minutes

Cooking Time: 9 minutes

Servings: 4

Ingredients:

- 1 tsp. fresh ginger, grated
- 2 medium garlic cloves, minced
- 1/4 cup coconut aminos
- 2 tbsp. fresh lime juice
- 1 ½ pound NY strip steak, trimmed and sliced thinly
- 2 medium zucchinis, spiralized with blade C
- Salt to taste
- 3 tbsp. essential olive oil
- 2 medium scallions, sliced
- 1 tsp. red pepper flakes, crushed
- 2 tbsp. fresh cilantro, chopped

Directions:

1. In a big bowl, merge ginger, garlic, coconut aminos, and lime juice. Add the beef and coat with the marinade generously. Refrigerate to soak for approximately 10 minutes.
2. Set zucchini noodles over a large paper towel and sprinkle with salt.
3. Keep aside for around 10 minutes.
4. In a big skillet, heat oil on medium-high heat. Attach the scallions, and red pepper flakes, then saute for about 1 minute.

5. Attach the beef with the marinade and stir fry for around 3–4 minutes or till browned.
6. Stir in the fresh cilantro, then add the zucchini and cook for approximately 3–4 minutes.
7. Serve hot.

Nutrition:

- Calories: 1366 kcal
- Carbs: 166 g
- Cholesterol: 6 mg
- Fat: 67 g
- Protein: 59 g
- Fiber. 41 g

66. Spiced Ground Beef

Preparation Time: 10 minutes

Cooking Time: 15 minutes

Servings: 5

Ingredients:

- 2 tbsp. coconut oil
- 2 whole cloves
- 2 whole cardamoms
- 1 (2 inches) piece cinnamon stick
- 2 bay leaves
- 1 tsp. cumin seeds
- 2 onions, chopped
- Salt to taste
- 1/2 tbsp. garlic paste
- 1/2 tbsp. fresh ginger paste
- 1 pound lean ground beef
- 1 ½ tsp. fennel seeds powder
- 1 tsp. ground cumin
- 1 ½ tsp. red chili powder
- 1/8 tsp. ground turmeric
- Freshly ground black pepper, to taste
- 1 cup coconut milk
- 1/4 cup water
- 1/4 cup fresh cilantro, chopped

Directions:

1. In a sizable pan, warm oil on medium heat. Mix cloves, cardamoms, cinnamon sticks, bay leaves, and cumin seeds; cook for about 20 seconds.
2. Attach the onion, and 2 pinches of salt, then saute for about 3–4 minutes.
3. Add the garlic-ginger paste and stir fry for about 2 minutes.
4. Attach the beef and cook for about 4–5 minutes, entering pieces using the spoon. Stir in spices and cook.
5. Set in the coconut milk and water; cook for about 3–4 minutes. Flavor with salt and take away from the heat.
6. Serve hot using the garnishing of cilantro.

Nutrition:

- Calories: 216 kcal
- Protein: 8.83 g
- Fat: 11.48 g
- Carbs: 21.86 g

67. Ground Beef with Veggies

Preparation Time: 60 minutes

Cooking Time: 15 minutes

Servings: 4

Ingredients:

- 1–2 tbsp. coconut oil
- 1 red onion,
- 2 red jalapeño peppers
- 2 minced garlic cloves
- 1 pound lean ground beef
- 1 small head broccoli, chopped
- 1/2 head cauliflower
- 3 carrots, peeled and sliced
- 3 celery ribs
- Chopped fresh thyme, to taste
- Dried sage, to taste
- Ground turmeric, to taste
- Salt and freshly ground black pepper

Directions:

1. In a large skillet, dissolve the coconut oil on medium heat.

2. Stir in the onion, jalapeño peppers, and garlic. Saute for about 5 minutes.
3. Attach the beef and cook for around 4–5 minutes, entering pieces using the spoon.
4. Add the remaining ingredients and cook, occasionally stirring for about 5 minutes.
5. Serve hot.

Nutrition:

- Calories: 141 kcal
- Cholesterol: 50 mg
- Carbs: 6 g
- Fat: 1 g
- Sugar: 3 g
- Fiber: 2 g

68. Ground Beef with Greens and Tomatoes

Preparation Time: 15 minutes

Cooking Time: 15 minutes

Servings: 4

Ingredients:

- 1 tbsp. organic olive oil
- 1/2 white onion, chopped
- 2 garlic cloves, finely chopped
- 1 jalapeño pepper, finely chopped
- 1 pound lean ground beef
- 1 tsp. ground coriander
- 1 tsp. ground cumin
- 1/2 tsp. ground turmeric
- 1/2 tsp. ground ginger
- 1/2 tsp. ground cinnamon
- 1/2 tsp. ground fennel seeds
- Salt and freshly ground black pepper
- 8 fresh cherry tomatoes, quartered
- 8 collard green leaves, stemmed and chopped
- 1 tsp. fresh lemon juice

Directions:

1. In a big skillet, warm oil on medium heat.
2. Add the onion and saute for approximately 4 minutes.
3. Stir in the garlic and jalapeño pepper. Saute for approximately 1 minute.
4. Attach the beef and spices; cook for approximately 6 minutes, breaking into pieces while using a spoon.
5. Set in tomatoes and greens. Cook, stirring gently for about 4 minutes.
6. Whisk in lemon juice and take away from the heat.

Nutrition:

- Calories: 444 kcal
- Fat: 15 g
- Carbs: 20 g
- Fiber: 2 g
- Protein: 37 g

69. Guacamole

Preparation Time: 10 minutes

Cooking Time: 0 minutes

Servings: 3

Ingredients:

- 3 ripe avocados
- 2 large tomatoes
- 2 tbsp. lemon juice
- 1 dash chili sauce (optional)
- 1/2 onion, chopped
- 1 large garlic clove, minced
- Sea salt and pepper

Directions:

1. Peel the avocados and mix the meat with lemon juice, onion, garlic, tomatoes, sea salt, pepper, and chili sauce well.
2. Serve with whole-grain tortillas and/or raw oven vegetables.

Nutrition:

- Calories: 35 kcal
- Fat: 0 g
- Carbs: 17 g
- Fiber: 0 g

- Protein: 0 g

70. Dark Chocolate with Pomegranate Seeds

Preparation Time: 10 minutes

Cooking Time: 2–3 minutes

Servings: 3

Ingredients:

- 150 g dark chocolate (at least 70% cocoa)
- 120 g pomegranate seeds (from 1 pomegranate)
- 1 tsp. sea salt

Directions:

1. Scatter a layer of pomegranate seeds in a muffin tin (or muffin paper).
2. Melt the chocolate in the microwave.
3. Pour the chocolate into a bag, then cut a tiny hole so that it can be spread over the seeds. Add a layer of seeds and another of chocolate.
4. Sprinkle with a pinch of salt and chill in the refrigerator until the mixture is hard.
5. Enjoy cold.

Nutrition:

- Calories: 82 kcal
- Carbs: 19 g
- Protein: 1.9 g
- Fat: 0.2 g
- Sugar: 3.9 g
- Sodium: 37 mg
- Fiber: 3.7 g

71. Covered Bananas

Preparation Time: 10 minutes

Cooking Time: 0 minutes

Servings: 3

Ingredients:

- 3 bananas
- 1 tbsp. oat bran
- 2 tbsp. cashew or almond butter
- 1 tbsp. honey
- 1 tsp. chia seeds
- 1 tsp. cinnamon

Directions:

1. Mix the oat bran, seeds, and cinnamon in a shallow bowl.
2. Mix the nut butter with honey.
3. Coat the bananas with nut butter and then add to the dry mixture so that they are coated on both sides.

Nutrition:

- Calories: 11 kcal
- Carbs: 3 g
- Protein: 0 g
- Fat: 0 g
- Sugar: 2.9 g
- Sodium: 0 mg
- Fiber: 0.1 g

72. Hummus with Tahini and Turmeric

Preparation Time: 10 minutes

Cooking Time: 0 minutes

Servings: 4

Ingredients:

- 2 cans chickpeas, drained
- 50 ml lemon juice
- 60 ml tahini
- 1 garlic clove, minced
- 2 tbsp. extra-virgin olive oil
- 1/2 tbsp. turmeric powder
- 1/2 tsp. sea salt

Directions:

1. Mix the tahini and lemon juice with olive oil, garlic, turmeric, and salt for about 30 seconds using a hand blender or kitchen utensil.
2. Add the chickpeas and puree, making sure that no chickpeas remain unmixed

on the sides. Pound until a uniform mixture is obtained.
3. Garnish with paprika powder and enjoy with any snacks, such as vegetable sticks.

Nutrition:

- Calories: 33 kcal
- Carbs: 8.1 g
- Protein: 0.2 g
- Fat: 0.1 g
- Sugar: 7.6 g
- Sodium: 130 mg
- Fiber: 0.1 g

73. Fiber Bars

Preparation Time: 10 minutes

Cooking Time: 15 minutes

Servings: 4

Ingredients:

- 120 g dried dates
- 120 g nuts (cashew, hazel, walnuts)

Directions:

1. Remove the date kernels and mash the fruits with a fork.
2. Chop the nuts in a blender, but they must not get the consistency of flour.
3. Mix the 2 together.
4. Form small "snakes" and flatten them lightly with a fork so that they get the shape of a bar.

Nutrition:

- Calories: 140 kcal
- Carbs: 0.6 g
- Protein: 25 g
- Fat: 2.6 g
- Sugar: 0.1 g
- Sodium: 73 mg

74. Roasted Carrot Sticks in a Honey Garlic Marinade

Preparation Time: 10 minutes

Cooking Time: 15 minutes

Servings: 4

Ingredients:

- 1 carrots bunch, halved lengthways
- 2 garlic cloves, minced
- 1 tbsp. honey
- 1 tbsp. lemon juice (alternatively apple cider vinegar)
- 40 g butter
- 3 tbsp. parsley, chopped

Directions:

1. Place the halved carrots on baking paper.
2. For the marinade, first, melt the butter. Add the garlic, honey, and lemon/vinegar, mix well.
3. Set over the carrots so that they are all covered with the marinade.
4. Bake in the oven at 180ºC for about 15 minutes. Turn regularly.
5. Garnish with parsley and serve with herb quark or yogurt.

Nutrition:

- Calories: 216 kcal
- Fat: 1 g
- Carbs: 37 g
- Fiber: 4 g
- Protein: 8 g

75. Apple and Pistachio Salad on Spinach

Preparation Time: 10 minutes

Cooking Time: 5 minutes

Servings: 4

Ingredients:

- 1 ½ tbsp. butter

- 1 pack baby spinach
- 1 apple, diced small
- 1 tsp. ginger, grated
- 60 g pistachios
- 1 tbsp. mustard
- 40 g Ricotta cheese
- 1 tbsp. honey
- 1 tbsp. lemon juice
- Salt and pepper

Directions:

1. Dissolve the butter in the pan, add the apple pieces, honey, ginger, and mustard. Fry over medium heat until the apples are lightly caramelized for (about 3–5 minutes).
2. Wash the spinach and divide between 2 bowls. Place the apples on the salad, garnish with Ricotta, and season with a little lemon juice, pistachios, salt, and pepper as desired.

Nutrition:

- Calories: 37 kcal
- Fat: 1 g
- Carbs: 3 g
- Fiber: 0 g
- Protein: 4 g
- Sodium: 58 mg

76. Tomato Cashew Pesto

Preparation Time: 10 minutes

Cooking Time: 0 minutes

Servings: 4

Ingredients:

- 95 g dried tomatoes
- 50 g cashew nuts
- 2 garlic cloves, minced
- 5 tbsp. extra-virgin olive oil
- 1 tbsp. oregano
- Parmesan cheese (optional)
- Salt and pepper

Directions:

1. Puree the garlic, tomatoes, oregano, oil, and cashews with a hand blender until the mixture is even.
2. Mix with whole-wheat pasta and serve. Flavor to taste with salt and pepper, then garnish with Parmesan.

Nutrition:

- Calories: 29 kcal
- Fat: 1 g
- Carbs: 2 g
- Fiber: 1 g
- Protein: 1 g

77. Sweet Potato Aioli

Preparation Time: 10 minutes

Cooking Time: 15 minutes

Servings: 4

Ingredients:

- 1 sweet potato
- 3 tbsp. olive oil
- 1 tbsp. mayonnaise
- 2–3 garlic cloves
- 1 tbsp. parsley, chopped

Directions:

1. Bake the sweet potato in the oven until it is soft (about 15 minutes at 200ºC).
2. Set out of the oven, let cool down briefly, peel and mix with 1 tbsp. of mayonnaise, oil, garlic, and parsley (use a hand blender).

Nutrition:

- Calories: 75
- Carbs: 0.1 g
- Protein: 13.4 g
- Fat: 1.7 g
- Sugar: 0 g
- Sodium: 253 mg

78. Eggplant Paste

Preparation Time: 10 minutes

Cooking Time: 15 minutes

Servings: 4

Ingredients:

- 1 eggplant
- 2 tbsp. tahini
- 2 garlic cloves
- 1 tbsp. lemon juice
- A turmeric pinch
- 30 g black olives
- 1 tbsp. olive oil
- 1 tbsp. parsley, chopped
- Salt and pepper

Directions:

1. Grill the eggplant in the oven at 190ºC for at least 15 minutes (until it is soft!).
2. Let cool and remove the skin. Set the eggplant in a container and use a fork to mash the meat into a paste.
3. Add the tahini, garlic, turmeric, olives, olive oil, and lemon juice; mix well. Season to taste with salt and pepper.
4. Garnish with parsley.

Nutrition:

- Calories: 75 kcal
- Carbs: 0.1 g
- Protein: 13.4 g
- Fat: 1.7 g
- Sugar: 0 g
- Sodium: 253 mg

79. Catalan Style Spinach

Preparation Time: 10 minutes

Cooking Time: 5 minutes

Servings: 4

Ingredients:

- 200 g fresh spinach
- 2 garlic cloves
- 2 tbsp. cashew nuts
- 3 tbsp. raisins
- 2–3 tbsp. extra-virgin olive oil

Directions:

1. Warm the oil and fry the garlic over medium heat.
2. After 1–2 minutes add the cashews and raisins. Fry for another minute.
3. Add the spinach (do not boil!), stir well.
4. Serve with Goat cheese and wholemeal baguette.

Nutrition:

- Calories: 59 kcal
- Fat: 1 g
- Carbs: 14 g
- Fiber: 1 g
- Protein: 1 g
- Sodium: 304 mg

80. Energy Balls

Preparation Time: 10 minutes

Cooking Time: 0 minutes

Servings: 4

Ingredients:

- 120 g oat bran
- 80 ml honey
- 120 g coconut flakes (health food store, drugstore)
- 60 g choice nuts, ground
- 60 g chia seeds, ground
- 40 g dark chocolate, finely chopped
- 1 tsp. yeast flakes
- 1 tsp. sea salt

Directions:

1. Mix all ingredients well in a container. Let the chia seeds soak for a moment.
2. Set small balls and put them in the fridge for about 45 minutes.

Nutrition:

- Calories: 75 kcal
- Carbs: 0.1 g
- Protein: 13.4 g
- Fat: 1.7 g
- Sugar: 0 g

- Sodium: 253 mg
- Fiber: 0 g

Chapter 6. Low-Residue Recipes

81. Bright Red Juice

Preparation Time: 10 minutes

Cooking Time: 0 minutes

Servings: 3

Ingredients:

- 6 tomatoes
- 1 celery stalk
- ¼ C. filtered water
- A salt pinch and ground black pepper
- 2–3 ice cubes

Directions:

1. Place all the ingredients in a blender and pulse until well combined.
2. Through a cheesecloth-lined strainer, strain the juice and transfer into 3 glasses.
3. Serve immediately.

Nutrition:

- Calories: 62 kcal
- Carbs: 13.7 g
- Protein: 2.5 g
- Fat: 0.5 g
- Sugar: 8.6 g
- Sodium: 95 mg
- Fiber: 4 g

82. Enticing Fresh Juice

Preparation Time: 10 minutes

Cooking Time: 0 minutes

Servings: 2

Ingredients:

- 3 C. fresh spinach
- 3 C. fresh arugula
- 1 large carrot, peeled and chopped roughly
- 2 celery stalks
- 1 lemon
- 1 (1-inch) piece fresh ginger

Directions:

1. Add all ingredients into a juicer and extract the juice according to the manufacturer's method.
2. Through a cheesecloth-lined strainer, strain the juice and transfer into 2 glasses.
3. Serve immediately.

Nutrition:

- Calories: 36 kcal
- Carbs: 7.1 g
- Protein: 2.5 g
- Fat: 0.4 g
- Sugar: 2.8 g
- Sodium: 78 mg
- Fiber: 2.7g

83. Super-Food Scramble

Preparation Time: 10 minutes

Cooking Time: 7 minutes

Servings: 3

Ingredients:

- 2 C. fresh spinach, chopped finely
- 1 tbsp. olive oil
- Salt and freshly ground black pepper, to taste
- ½ C. cooked salmon, chopped finely
- 4 eggs, beaten

Directions:

1. In a skillet, heat the oil over high heat and cook the spinach with black pepper for about 2 minutes.
2. Stir in the salmon and reduce the heat to medium.
3. Add the eggs and cook for about 3–4 minutes, stirring frequently.
4. Serve immediately.

Nutrition:

- Calories: 179 kcal

- Carbs: 1.2 g
- Protein: 15.3 g
- Fat: 12.9 g
- Sugar: 0.5 g
- Sodium: 165 mg
- Fiber: 0.4 g

84. Family Favorite Scramble

Preparation Time: 10 minutes

Cooking Time: 5 minutes

Servings: 2

Ingredients:

- 4 eggs
- ¼ tsp. red pepper flakes, crushed
- Salt and freshly ground black pepper, to taste
- ¼ C. fresh basil, chopped
- ½ C. tomatoes, peeled, seeded, and chopped
- 1 tbsp. olive oil

Directions:

1. In a large bowl, add eggs, red pepper flakes, salt, and black pepper and beat well.
2. Add the basil and tomatoes and stir to combine.
3. In a large non-stick skillet, heat the oil over medium-high heat.
4. Add the egg mixture and cook for about 3–5 minutes, stirring continuously.
5. Serve immediately.

Nutrition:

- Calories: 195 kcal
- Carbs: 2.6 g
- Protein: 11.6 g
- Fat: 15.9 g
- Sugar: 1.9 g
- Sodium: 203 mg
- Fiber: 0.7 g

85. Tasty Veggie Omelet

Preparation Time: 15 minutes

Cooking Time: 15 minutes

Servings: 4

Ingredients:

- 6 large eggs
- Sea salt and freshly ground black pepper, to taste
- ½ C. low-fat milk
- 1/3 C. fresh mushrooms, cut into slices
- 1/3 C. red bell pepper, seeded and chopped
- 1 tbsp. chives, minced

Directions:

1. Preheat the oven to 350°F. Lightly, grease a pie dish.
2. In a bowl, add the eggs, salt, black pepper, and coconut oil and beat until well combined.
3. In another bowl, mix together the onion, bell pepper, and mushrooms.
4. Transfer the egg mixture into the prepared pie dish evenly.
5. Top with the vegetable mixture evenly and sprinkle with chives evenly.
6. Bake for about 15 minutes.
7. Remove from the oven and set aside for about 5 minutes.
8. With a knife, cut into equal-sized wedges and serve.

Nutrition:

- Calories: 125 kcal
- Carbs: 3.1 g
- Protein: 10.8 g
- Fat: 7.8 g
- Sugar: 2.8 g
- Sodium: 158 mg
- Fiber: 0.2 g

86. Garden Veggies Quiche

Preparation Time: 15 minutes

Cooking Time: 15 minutes

Servings: 4

Ingredients:

- 6 eggs
- ½ C. low-fat milk
- Salt and freshly ground black pepper, to taste
- 2 C. fresh baby spinach, chopped
- ½ C. green bell pepper, seeded and chopped
- 1 scallion, chopped
- ¼ C. fresh parsley, chopped
- 1 tbsp. fresh chives, minced

Directions:

1. Preheat the oven to 400°F. Lightly grease a pie dish.
2. In a bowl, add eggs, almond milk, salt, and black pepper and beat until well combined. Set aside.
3. In another bowl, add the vegetables and herbs and mix well.
4. In the bottom of the prepared pie dish, place the veggie mixture evenly and top with the egg mixture.
5. Bake for about 15 minutes or until a wooden skewer inserted in the center comes out clean.
6. Remove the pie dish from the oven and set it aside for about 5 minutes before slicing. Cut into desired-sized wedges and serve warm.

Nutrition:

- Calories: 118 kcal
- Carbs: 4.3 g
- Protein: 10.1 g
- Fat: 7 g
- Sugar: 3 g
- Sodium: 160 mg
- Fiber: 0.8 g

87. Stunning Breakfast Frittata

Preparation Time: 15 minutes

Cooking Time: 12 minutes

Servings: 6

Ingredients:

- 8 eggs, beaten well
- 8 tbsp. low-fat milk
- Salt and freshly ground black pepper, to taste
- 2 oz. feta cheese, crumbled
- ½ C. low-fat mozzarella cheese, grated
- ¼ C. scallion, sliced
- 2 tsp. olive oil
- 1 large avocado, peeled, pitted, and sliced lengthwise

Directions:

1. Preheat the broiler of the oven.
2. Arrange the oven rack about 4–5-inch from the heating element.
3. In a bowl, add the eggs, almond milk, salt, and black pepper and beat until well combined.
4. In a heavy oven-proof frying skillet, heat the oil over medium-low heat.
5. Add the eggs and cook for about 2 minutes.
6. Add the mozzarella and scallion and cook for about 5 minutes.
7. Arrange the avocado slices over the egg mixture and sprinkle with the feta cheese.
8. With a lid, cover the skillet and cook for about 3 minutes.
9. Remove the lid and transfer the skillet into the oven.
10. Broil for about 2 minutes.
11. Remove from the oven and serve hot.

Nutrition:

- Calories: 207 kcal
- Carbs: 5.1 g
- Protein: 10.8 g
- Fat: 16.6 g

- Sugar: 2.2 g
- Sodium: 241 mg
- Fiber: 2.4 g

88. Fluffy Pumpkin Pancakes

Preparation Time: 10 minutes

Cooking Time: 15 minutes

Servings: 10

Ingredients:

- 2 eggs
- 1 C. buckwheat flour
- 1 tbsp. baking powder
- 1 tsp. pumpkin pie spice
- ½ tsp. salt
- 1 C. pumpkin puree
- ¾ C. plus 2 tbsp. low-fat milk
- 3 tbsp. pure maple syrup
- 2 tbsp. olive oil
- 1 tsp. vanilla extract

Directions:

1. In a blender, add all ingredients and pulse until well combined.
2. Transfer the mixture into a bowl and set aside for about 10 minutes.
3. Heat a greased non-stick skillet over medium heat.
4. Place about ¼ C. of the mixture and spread in an even circle.
5. Cook for about 2 minutes per side.
6. Repeat with the remaining mixture.
7. Serve warm.

Nutrition:

- Calories: 113 kcal
- Carbs: 16.5 g
- Protein: 3.6 g
- Fat: 4.4 g
- Sugar: 5.9 g
- Sodium: 143 mg
- Fiber: 2 g

89. Super-Tasty Chicken Muffins

Preparation Time: 15 minutes

Cooking Time: 15 minutes

Servings: 8

Ingredients:

- 8 eggs
- Salt and freshly ground black pepper, as required
- 2 tbsp. filtered water
- 7 oz. cooked chicken, chopped finely
- 1½ C. fresh spinach, chopped
- 1 C. green bell pepper, seeded and chopped finely
- 2 tbsp. fresh parsley, chopped finely

Directions:

1. Preheat the oven to 350°F. Grease 8 C. of a muffin tin.
2. In a bowl, add eggs, salt, black pepper, and water and beat until well combined.
3. Add the chicken, spinach, bell pepper, and parsley and stir to combine.
4. Transfer the mixture into the prepared muffin C. evenly.
5. Bake for about 15 minutes or until golden brown.
6. Remove the muffin tin from the oven and place it onto a wire rack to cool for about 10 minutes.
7. Carefully invert the muffins onto a platter and serve warm.

Nutrition:

- Calories: 107
- Carbs: 1.7 g
- Protein: 13.1 g
- Fat: 5.2 g
- Sugar: 1.1 g
- Sodium: 102 mg
- Fiber: 0.4 g

90. Classic Zucchini Bread

Preparation Time: 45 minutes

Cooking Time: 15 minutes

Servings: 24

Ingredients:

- 3 C. all-purpose flour
- 2 tsp. baking soda
- 1 tsp. ground cinnamon
- 1 tsp. ground nutmeg
- 2 C. Splenda
- 1 C. olive oil
- 3 eggs, beaten
- 2 tsp. vanilla extract
- 2 C. zucchini, peeled, seeded, and grated

Directions:

1. Preheat the oven to 325°F. Arrange a rack in the center of the oven. Grease 2 loaf pans.
2. In a medium bowl, mix together the flour, baking soda, and spices.
3. In another large bowl, add the Splenda and oil and beat until well combined.
4. Add the eggs and vanilla extract and beat until well combined.
5. Add the flour mixture and mix until just combined.
6. Gently, fold in the zucchini.
7. Place the mixture into the bread loaf pans evenly.
8. Bake for about 45–50 minutes or until a toothpick inserted in the center of the bread comes out clean.
9. Remove the bread pans from the oven and place them onto a wire rack to cool for about 15 minutes.
10. Carefully, invert the bread onto the wire rack to cool completely before slicing.
11. With a sharp knife, cut each bread loaf into desired-sized slices and serve.

Nutrition:

- Calories: 219 kcal
- Carbs: 28.4 g
- Protein: 16.3 g
- Fat: 9.2 g
- Sugar: 16.3 g
- Sodium: 113 mg
- Fiber: 0.6 g

91. Greek Inspired Cucumber Salad

Preparation Time: 10 minutes

Servings: 4

Ingredients:

- 4 medium cucumbers, peeled, seeded, and chopped
- ½ C. low-fat Greek yogurt
- 1½ tbsp. fresh dill, chopped
- 1 tbsp. fresh lemon juice
- Salt and freshly ground black pepper, as required

Directions:

1. In a large bowl, add all the ingredients and mix well.
2. Serve immediately.

Nutrition:

- Calories: 71 kcal
- Carbs: 13.8 g
- Protein: 4 g
- Fat: 0.8 g
- Sugar: 7.3 g
- Sodium: 69 mg
- Fiber: 1.7 g

92. Light Veggie Salad

Preparation Time: 10 minutes

Servings: 5

Ingredients:

- 2 C. cucumbers, peeled, seeded, and chopped
- 2 C. red tomatoes, peeled, seeded, and chopped
- 2 tbsp. extra-virgin olive oil
- 2 tbsp. fresh lime juice

- Salt, to taste

Directions:

1. In a large serving bowl, add all the ingredients and toss to coat well.
2. Serve immediately.

Nutrition:

- Calories: 68 kcal
- Carbs: 04.4 g
- Protein: 0.9 g
- Fat: 5.8 g
- Sugar: 2.6 g
- Sodium: 35 mg
- Fiber: 1.1 g

93. Eastern European Soup

Preparation Time: 10 minutes

Cooking Time: 5 minutes

Servings: 3

Ingredients:

- 2 C. fat-free yogurt
- 4 tsp. fresh lemon juice
- 2 C. beets, trimmed, peeled, and chopped
- 2 tbsp. fresh dill
- Salt, as required
- 1 tbsp. fresh chives, minced

Directions:

1. In a high-speed blender, add all ingredients except for chives and pulse until smooth.
2. Transfer the soup into a pan over medium heat and cook for about 3–5 minutes or until heated through.
3. Serve immediately with the garnishing of chives.

Nutrition:

- Calories: 149 kcal
- Carbs: 25.2 g
- Protein: 11.8 g
- Fat: 0.6 g
- Sugar: 21.7 g
- Sodium: 269 mg
- Fiber: 2.5g

94. Citrus Glazed Carrots

Preparation Time: 15 minutes

Cooking Time: 15 minutes

Servings: 6

Ingredients:

- 1½ lb. carrots, peeled and sliced into ½-inch pieces diagonally
- ½ C. water
- 2 tbsp. olive oil
- Salt, to taste
- 3 tbsp. fresh orange juice

Directions:

1. In a large skillet, add the carrots, water, boil, and salt over medium heat and bring to a boil.
2. Reduce heat to low and simmer; covered for about 6 minutes.
3. Add the orange juice and stir to combine.
4. Increase the heat to high and cook, uncovered for about 5–8 minutes, tossing frequently.
5. Serve immediately.

Nutrition:

- Calories: 90 kcal
- Carbs: 12 g
- Protein: 1 g
- Fat: 4.7 g
- Sugar: 6.2 g
- Sodium: 106 mg
- Fiber: 2.8 g

95. Braised Asparagus

Preparation Time: 10 minutes

Cooking Time: 8 minutes

Servings: 2

Ingredients:

- ½ C. chicken bone broth
- 1 tbsp. olive oil
- 1 (½-inch) lemon peel
- 1 C. asparagus, trimmed

Directions:

1. In a small pan, add the broth, oil, and lemon peel over medium heat and bring to a boil.
2. Add the asparagus and cook, covered for about 3–4 minutes.
3. Discard the lemon peel and serve.

Nutrition:

- Calories: 82 kcal
- Carbs: 2.6 g
- Protein: 3.7 g
- Fat: 7.1 g
- Sugar: 1.3 g
- Sodium: 25 mg
- Fiber: 1.4 g

96. Spring Flavored Pasta

Preparation Time: 10 minutes

Cooking Time: 10 minutes

Servings: 4

Ingredients:

- 2 tbsp. olive oil
- 1 lb. asparagus, trimmed and cut into 1½-inch pieces
- Salt and freshly ground black pepper, to taste
- ½ lb. cooked hot pasta, drained

Directions:

1. In a large cast-iron skillet, heat the oil over medium heat and cook the asparagus, salt, and black pepper for about 8–10 minutes, stirring occasionally.
2. Place the hot pasta and toss to coat well.
3. Serve immediately.

Nutrition:

- Calories: 246 kcal
- Carbs: 35.2 g
- Protein: 8.9 g
- Fat: 8.4 g
- Sugar: 2.1 g
- Sodium: 17 mg
- Fiber: 2.4 g

97. Versatile Mac 'n Cheese

Preparation Time: 15 minutes

Cooking Time: 12 minutes

Servings: 2

Ingredients:

- 2 C. elbow macaroni
- 1½ s butternut squash, peeled and cubed
- 1 C. low-fat Swiss cheese, shredded
- 1/3 C. low-fat milk
- 1 tbsp. olive oil
- Salt and freshly ground black pepper, to taste

Directions:

1. In a large pan of the salted boiling water, cook the macaroni for about 8–10 minutes.
2. Drain the macaroni and transfer it into a bowl.
3. Meanwhile, cook the squash cubes for about 6 minutes or until soft in a pan of boiling water.
4. Drain the squash cubes completely and return to the same pan.
5. With a masher, mash the squash and place over low heat.
6. Add the cheese and milk and cook for about 2–3 minutes, stirring continuously.
7. Add the macaroni, oil, salt, and black pepper and stir to combine.
8. Remove from the heat and serve hot.

Nutrition:

- Calories: 321 kcal
- Carbs: 40 g

- Protein: 14 g
- Fat: 11.9 g
- Sugar: 3.7 g
- Sodium: 65 mg
- Fiber: 2.4 g

98. Gluten-Free Curry

Preparation Time: 15 minutes

Cooking Time: 20 minutes

Servings: 6

Ingredients:

- 2 C. tomatoes, peeled, seeded, and chopped
- 1½ C. water
- 2 tbsp. olive oil
- 1 tsp. fresh ginger, chopped
- ¼ tsp. ground turmeric
- 2 C. fresh shiitake mushrooms, sliced
- 5 C. fresh button mushrooms, sliced
- ¼ C. fat-free yogurt, whipped
- Salt and freshly ground black pepper, to taste

Directions:

1. In a food processor, add the tomatoes and ¼ C. of water and pulse until smooth paste forms.
2. In a pan, heat the oil over medium heat and sauté the ginger and turmeric for about 1 minute.
3. Add the tomato paste and cook for about 5 minutes.
4. Stir in the mushrooms, yogurt, and remaining water and bring to a boil.
5. Cook for about 10–12 minutes, stirring occasionally.
6. Season with salt and black pepper and remove from the heat.
7. Serve hot.

Nutrition:

- Calories: 70 kcal
- Carbs: 5.3 g
- Protein: 3 g
- Fat: 5 g
- Sugar: 3.4 g
- Sodium: 41 mg
- Fiber: 1.4 g

99. New Year's Luncheon Meal

Preparation Time: 10 minutes

Servings: 2

Ingredients:

- 1 large avocado, halved and pitted
- 1 (5-oz.) can water-packed tuna, drained and flaked
- 3 tbsp. fat-free yogurt
- 2 tbsp. fresh lemon juice
- 1 tsp. fresh parsley, chopped finely
- Salt and freshly ground black pepper, to taste

Directions:

1. Carefully, remove abut about 2–3 tbsp. of flesh from each avocado half.
2. Arrange the avocado halves onto a platter and drizzle each with 1 tsp. of lemon juice.
3. Chop the avocado flesh and transfer into a bowl.
4. In the bowl of avocado flesh, add tuna, yogurt, parsley, remaining lemon juice, salt, and black pepper, and stir to combine.
5. Divide the tuna mixture into both avocado halves evenly.
6. Serve immediately.

Nutrition:

- Calories: 215 kcal
- Carbs: 7 g
- Protein: 20.6 g
- Fat: 11.8 g
- Sugar: 2.4 g
- Sodium: 137 mg
- Fiber: 3.2 g

100. Entertaining Wraps

Preparation Time: 15 minutes

Cooking Time: 10 minutes

Servings: 5

Ingredients:

For Chicken:

- 2 tbsp. olive oil
- 1 tsp. fresh ginger, minced
- 1¼ lb. ground chicken
- Salt and freshly ground black pepper, to taste

For Wraps:

- 10 romaine lettuce leaves
- 1½ C. carrot, peeled and julienned
- 2 tbsp. fresh parsley, chopped finely
- 2 tbsp. fresh lime juice

Directions:

1. In a skillet, heat the oil over medium heat and sauté the ginger for about 1 minute.
2. Add the ground chicken, salt, and black pepper and cook for about 7–9 minutes, breaking up the meat into smaller pieces with a wooden spoon.
3. Remove from the heat and set aside to cool.
4. Arrange the lettuce leaves onto serving plates.
5. Place the cooked chicken over each lettuce leaf and top with carrot and cilantro.
6. Drizzle with lime juice and serve immediately.

Nutrition:

- Calories: 280 kcal
- Carbs: 3.8 g
- Protein: 33.2 g
- Fat: 14 g
- Sugar: 1.7 g
- Sodium: 153 mg
- Fiber: 0.9 g

101. Outdoor Chicken Kabobs

Preparation Time: 15 minutes

Cooking Time: 7 minutes

Servings: 4

Ingredients:

- ¼ C. low-fat Parmesan cheese, grated
- 3 tbsp. olive oil
- 1 C. fresh basil leaves, chopped
- Salt and freshly ground black pepper, to taste
- 1¼ lb. boneless, skinless chicken breast, cut into 1-inch cubes

Directions:

1. In a food processor, add the cheese, oil, garlic, basil, salt, and black pepper, and pulse until smooth.
2. Transfer the basil mixture into a large bowl.
3. Add the chicken cubes and mix well.
4. Cover the bowl and refrigerate to marinate for at least 4–5 hours.
5. Preheat the grill to medium-high heat. Generously, grease the grill grate.
6. Thread the chicken cubes onto pre-soaked wooden skewers.
7. Place the skewers onto the grill and cook for about 3–4 minutes.
8. Flip and cook for about 2-3 minutes more.
9. Remove from the grill and place onto a platter for about 5 minutes before serving.
10. Serve hot.

Nutrition:

- Calories: 270 kcal
- Carbs: 0.3 g
- Protein: 31.5 g
- Fat: 15.3 g
- Sugar: 0 g
- Sodium: 207 mg
- Fiber: 0.1 g

102. Flavorful Shrimp Kabobs

Preparation Time: 15 minutes

Cooking Time: 8 minutes

Servings: 4

Ingredients:

- ¼ C. olive oil
- 2 tbsp. fresh lime juice
- 1 tsp. honey
- ½ tsp. paprika
- ¼ tsp. ground cumin
- Salt and freshly ground black pepper, to taste
- 1 lb. medium raw shrimp, peeled and deveined

Directions:

1. In a large bowl, add all the ingredients except for shrimp and mix well.
2. Add the shrimp and coat with the herb mixture generously.
3. Refrigerate to marinate for at least 30 minutes.
4. Preheat the grill to medium-high heat. Grease the grill grate.
5. Thread the shrimp onto pre-soaked wooden skewers.
6. Place the skewers onto the grill and cook for about 2–4 minutes per side.
7. Remove from the grill and place onto a platter for about 5 minutes before serving.

Nutrition:

- Calories: 250 kcal
- Carbs: 3.4 g
- Protein: 25.9 g
- Fat: 14.6 g
- Sugar: 01.5 g
- Sodium: 316 mg
- Fiber: 0.1 g

103. Pan-Seared Scallops

Preparation Time: 15 minutes

Cooking Time: 7 minutes

Servings: 4

Ingredients:

- 1¼ lb. fresh sea scallops, side muscles removed
- Salt and freshly ground black pepper, to taste
- 2 tbsp. olive oil
- 1 tbsp. fresh parsley, minced

Directions:

1. Sprinkle the scallops with salt and black pepper.
2. In a large skillet, heat the oil over medium-high heat and cook the scallops for about 2–3 minutes per side.
3. Stir in the parsley and remove from the heat.
4. Serve hot.

Nutrition:

- Calories: 185 kcal
- Carbs: 3.4 g
- Protein: 23.8 g
- Fat: 8.1 g
- Sugar: 0 g
- Sodium: 268 mg
- Fiber: 0 g

104. Mediterranean Shrimp Salad

Preparation Time: 15 minutes

Cooking Time: 3 minutes

Servings: 5

Ingredients:

- 1 lb. shrimp, peeled and deveined
- 1 lemon, quartered
- 2 tbsp. olive oil
- 2 tsp. fresh lemon juice
- Salt and freshly ground black pepper, to taste

- 3 tomatoes, peeled, seeded, and sliced
- ¼ C. olives, pitted
- ¼ C. fresh cilantro, chopped finely

Directions:

1. In a pan of lightly salted water, add the quartered lemon and bring to a boil.
2. Add the shrimp and cook for about 2–3 minutes or until pink and opaque.
3. With a slotted spoon, transfer the shrimp into a bowl of ice water to stop the cooking process.
4. Drain the shrimp completely, and then pat dry with paper towels.
5. In a small bowl, add the oil, lemon juice, salt, and black pepper, and beat until well combined.
6. Divide the shrimp, tomato, olives, and cilantro onto serving plates.
7. Drizzle with oil mixture and serve.

Nutrition:

- Calories: 178 kcal
- Carbs: 5 g
- Protein: 21.4 g
- Fat: 8 g
- Sugar: 2.1 g
- Sodium: 315 mg
- Fiber: 1.2 g

105. Health Conscious People's Salad

Preparation Time: 15 minutes

Servings: 2

Ingredients:

- ¼ C. low-fat mozzarella cheese, cubed
- ¼ C. tomato, peeled, seeded, and chopped
- 1 tbsp. fresh dill, chopped
- 1 tsp. fresh lemon juice
- Salt, to taste
- 6 oz. cooked salmon, chopped

Directions:

1. In a small bowl, add all the ingredients and stir to combine.
2. Serve immediately.

Nutrition:

- Calories: 131 kcal
- Carbs: 1.9 g
- Protein: 18 g
- Fat: 6 g
- Sugar: 0.6 g
- Sodium: 141 mg
- Fiber: 0.5 g

106. Italian Pasta Soup

Preparation Time: 15 minutes

Cooking Time: 15 minutes

Servings: 5

Ingredients:

- 1 potato, peeled and chopped
- 1 carrot, peeled and chopped
- 5¼ C. chicken bone broth
- ½ C. tomato, peeled, seeded, and chopped
- ¾ lb. asparagus tips
- ½ C. cooked small pasta
- Salt and freshly ground black pepper, to taste

Directions:

1. In a pan, add the potato, carrot, and broth over medium-high heat and bring to a boil.
2. Reduce the heat to low and cook, covered for about 8 minutes or until vegetables become tender.
3. Add the tomatoes and asparagus and cook for about 4–5 minutes.
4. Stir in the cooked pasta, salt, and black pepper and cook for about 2–3 minutes.
5. Serve hot.

Nutrition:

- Calories: 147 kcal
- Carbs: 23.2 g

- Protein: 13.6 g
- Fat: 0.5 g
- Sugar: 3.5 g
- Sodium: 108 mg
- Fiber: 3 g

107. Pure Comfort Soup

Preparation Time: 10 minutes

Cooking Time: 15 minutes

Servings: 4

Ingredients:

- 6 C. chicken bone broth
- 1/3 C. orzo
- 6 large egg yolks
- 1½ C. cooked chicken, shredded
- ¼ C. fresh lemon juice
- Salt and freshly ground black pepper, to taste

Directions:

1. In a large pan, add the broth over medium-high heat and bring to a boil.
2. Add the pasta and cook for about 6–7 minutes.
3. In a slowly, add in 1 C. of the hot broth, beating continuously.
4. Add the egg mixture to the pan, stirring continuously.
5. Reduce the heat to medium and cook for about 5–6 minutes, frequently stirring.
6. Stir in the cooked chicken, salt, and black pepper and cook for about 1–2 minutes.
7. Remove from the heat and serve hot.

Nutrition:

- Calories: 269 kcal
- Carbs: 11.9 g
- Protein: 34.6 g
- Fat: 8.7 g
- Sugar: 1.2 g
- Sodium: 230 mg
- Fiber: 0.6 g

108. Good-for-You Stew

Preparation Time: 15 minutes

Cooking Time: 15 minutes

Servings: 8

Ingredients:

- 2½ C. fresh tomatoes, peeled, seeded, and chopped
- 4 C. fish bone broth
- 1 lb. salmon fillets, cubed
- 1 lb. shrimp, peeled and deveined
- 2 tbsp. fresh lime juice
- Salt and freshly ground black pepper, to taste
- 3 tbsp. fresh parsley, chopped

Directions:

1. In a large soup pan, add the tomatoes and broth and bring to a boil.
2. Reduce the heat to medium and simmer for about 5 minutes.
3. Add the salmon and simmer for about 3–4 minutes.
4. Stir in the shrimp and cook for about 4–5 minutes.
5. Stir in lemon juice, salt, and black pepper, and remove from heat.
6. Serve hot with the garnishing of parsley.

Nutrition:

- Calories: 173 kcal
- Carbs: 3.2 g
- Protein: 27.1 g
- Fat: 5.5 g
- Sugar: 1.5 g
- Sodium: 368 mg
- Fiber: 0.7 g

109. Zero-Fiber Chicken Dish

Preparation Time: 16 minutes

Cooking Time: 10 minutes

Servings: 6

Ingredients:

- 4 (6-oz.) boneless, skinless chicken breast halves
- Salt and freshly ground black pepper, to taste
- 2 tbsp. olive oil

Directions:

1. Season each chicken breast half with salt and black pepper evenly.
2. Place chicken breast halves over a rack set in a rimmed baking sheet.
3. Refrigerate for at least 30 minutes.
4. Remove from refrigerator and pat dry with paper towels.
5. In a skillet, heat the oil over medium-low heat.
6. Place the chicken breast halves, smooth-side down, and cook for about 9–10 minutes, without moving.
7. Flip the chicken breasts and cook for about 6 minutes or until cooked through.
8. Remove from the heat and let the chicken stand in the pan for about 3 minutes.
9. Now, place the chicken breasts onto a cutting board.
10. Cut each chicken breast into slices and serve.

Nutrition:

- Calories: 255 kcal
- Carbs: 0 g
- Protein: 32.8 g
- Fat: 13.1 g
- Sugar: 0 g
- Sodium: 125 mg
- Fiber: 0 g

110. Amazing Chicken Platter

Preparation Time: 15 minutes

Cooking Time: 15 minutes

Servings: 6

Ingredients:

- 2 tbsp. olive oil, divided
- 4 (4-oz.) boneless, skinless chicken breasts, cut into small pieces
- Salt and freshly ground black pepper, to taste
- 1 tsp. fresh ginger, grated
- 4 C. fresh mushrooms, sliced
- 1 C. chicken bone broth

Directions:

1. In a large skillet, heat 1 tbsp. of oil over medium-high heat and stir fry the chicken pieces, salt, and black pepper for about 4–5 minutes or until golden brown.
2. With a slotted spoon, transfer the chicken pieces onto a plate.
3. In the same skillet, heat the remaining oil over medium heat and sauté the onion, ginger for about 1 minute.
4. Add the mushrooms and cook for about 4–5 minutes, stirring frequently.
5. Add the cooked chicken and coconut milk and stir fry for about 3–4 minutes
6. Add in the salt and black pepper and remove from the heat.
7. Serve hot.

Nutrition:

- Calories: 200 kcal
- Carbs: 1.6 g
- Protein: 24.8 g
- Fat: 10.4 g
- Sugar: 0.8 g
- Sodium: 111 mg
- Fiber: 0.5 g

111. Colorful Chicken Dinner

Preparation Time: 15 minutes

Cooking Time: 15 minutes

Servings: 6

Ingredients:

- 3 tbsp. olive oil, divided
- 1 large yellow bell pepper, seeded and sliced
- 1 large red bell pepper, seeded and sliced
- 1 large green bell pepper, seeded and sliced
- 1 lb. boneless, skinless chicken breasts, sliced thinly
- 1 tsp. dried oregano, crushed
- ¼ tsp. garlic powder
- ¼ tsp. ground cumin
- Salt and freshly ground black pepper, to taste
- ¼ C. chicken bone broth

Directions:

1. In a skillet, heat 1 tbsp. of oil over medium-high heat and cook the bell peppers for about 4–5 minutes.
2. With a slotted spoon, transfer the peppers mixture onto a plate.
3. In the same skillet, heat the remaining over medium-high heat and cook the chicken for about 6 minutes, stirring frequently.
4. Stir in the thyme, spices, salt, black pepper, and broth, and bring to a boil.
5. Add the peppers mixture and stir to combine.
6. Reduce the heat to medium and cook for about 3–4 minutes or until all the liquid is absorbed, stirring occasionally. Serve immediately.

Nutrition:

- Calories: 226 kcal
- Carbs: 4.8 g
- Protein: 22.9 g
- Fat: 12.8 g
- Sugar: 3 g
- Sodium: 98 mg
- Fiber: 0.9 g

112. Easiest Tuna Salad

Preparation Time: 15 minutes

Servings: 4

Ingredients:

For Dressing:

- 2 tbsp. fresh dill, minced
- 2 tbsp. olive oil
- 1 tbsp. fresh lime juice
- Salt and freshly ground black pepper, to taste

For Salad:

- 2 (6-oz.) cans water-packed tuna, drained and flaked
- 6 hard-boiled eggs, peeled and sliced
- 1 C. tomato, peeled, seeded, and chopped
- 1 large cucumber, peeled, seeded, and sliced

Directions:

For dressing:

1. In a small bowl, add all the ingredients and beat until well combined.

For salad:

1. In another large serving bowl, add all the ingredients and mix well.
2. Divide the tuna mixture onto serving plates.
3. Drizzle with dressing and serve.

Nutrition:

- Calories: 277 kcal
- Carbs: 5.9 g
- Protein: 31.2 g
- Fat: 14.5 g
- Sugar: 3 g
- Sodium: 181 mg
- Fiber: 1.1 g

113. Lemony Salmon

Preparation Time: 10 minutes

Cooking Time: 14 minutes

Servings: 4

Ingredients:

- 1 tbsp. fresh lemon zest, grated
- 2 tbsp. extra-virgin olive oil
- 2 tbsp. fresh lemon juice
- Salt and freshly ground black pepper, to taste
- 4 (6-oz.) boneless, skinless salmon fillets

Directions:

1. Preheat the grill to medium-high heat. Grease the grill grate.
2. In a bowl, place all ingredients except for salmon fillets and mix well.
3. Add the salmon fillets and coat with garlic mixture generously.
4. Place the salmon fillets onto the grill and cook for about 6–7 minutes per side.
5. Serve hot.

Nutrition:

- Calories: 290 kcal
- Carbs: 1 g
- Protein: 33.2 g
- Fat: 21.5 g
- Sugar: 0.3 g
- Sodium: 116 mg
- Fiber: 0.2 g

114. Herbed Salmon

Preparation Time: 10 minutes

Cooking Time: 8 minutes

Servings: 4

Ingredients:

- 1 tsp. dried oregano, crushed
- 1 tsp. dried basil, crushed
- Salt and freshly ground black pepper, to taste
- ¼ C. olive oil
- 2 tbsp. fresh lemon juice
- 4 (4-oz.) salmon fillets

Directions:

1. In a large bowl, add all ingredients except for salmon and mix well.
2. Add the salmon and coat with marinade generously.
3. Cover the bowl and refrigerate to marinate for at least 1 hour.
4. Preheat the grill to medium-high heat. Grease the grill grate.
5. Place the salmon onto the grill and cook for about 4 minutes per side.
6. Serve hot.

Nutrition:

- Calories: 261 kcal
- Carbs: 0.4 g
- Protein: 22.1 g
- Fat: 19.7 g
- Sugar: 0.2 g
- Sodium: 80 mg
- Fiber: 0.2 g

115. Delicious Combo Dinner

Preparation Time: 15 minutes

Cooking Time: 15 minutes

Servings: 5

Ingredients:

- 2 tbsp. olive oil
- 1 lb. prawns, peeled and deveined
- 1 lb. asparagus, trimmed
- Salt and freshly ground black pepper, to taste
- 1 tsp. fresh ginger, minced
- 2 tbsp. fresh lemon juice

Directions:

1. In a skillet, heat 1 tbsp. of oil over medium-high heat and cook the prawns with salt and black pepper for about 3–4 minutes.

2. With a slotted spoon, transfer the prawns into a bowl. Set aside.
3. In the same skillet, heat the remaining oil over medium-high heat and cook the asparagus, ginger, salt, and black pepper for about 6–8 minutes, stirring frequently.
4. Stir in the prawns and cook for about 1 minute.
5. Stir in the lemon juice and remove from the heat.
6. Serve hot.

Nutrition:

- Calories: 176 kcal
- Carbs: 5.1 g
- Protein: 22.7 g
- Fat: 7.3 g
- Sugar: 1.9 g
- Sodium: 255 mg
- Fiber: 1.9 g

116. Chicken Cutlets

Preparation Time: 10 minutes

Cooking Time: 15 minutes

Servings: 4

Ingredients:

- 4 tsp. red wine vinegar
- 2 tsp. minced garlic cloves
- 2 tsp. dried sage leaves
- 1 pound chicken breast cutlets
- Salt and pepper, to taste
- 1/4 cup refined white flour
- 2 tsp. olive oil

Directions:

1. Set a good amount of plastic wrap on the kitchen counter; sprinkle with half the combined sage, garlic, and vinegar.
2. Put the chicken breast on the plastic wrap; sprinkle with the rest of the vinegar mixture. Season lightly with pepper and salt.
3. Secure the chicken with the second sheet of plastic wrap. Use a kitchen mallet to pound the breast until it is flattened. Let stand 5 minutes.
4. Set the chicken on both sides with flour. In a skillet, heat the oil over medium heat.
5. Add half of the chicken breast and cook for 1 ½ minute or until it is browned on the bottom.
6. Turn on the other side and let it cook for 3 minutes.
7. Remove the chicken breast and place it on an oven-proof serving plate so that you can keep warm.
8. Reduce the liquid by half. Pour the mixture over the chicken breast; serve immediately.

Nutrition:

- Calories: 549 kcal
- Fat: 6 g
- Carbs: 7 g
- Fiber: 1 g
- Protein: 114 g

117. Salsa Turkey

Preparation Time: 8 minutes

Cooking Time: 15 minutes

Servings: 4

Ingredients:

- 2 pounds turkey breasts, boneless and skinless
- 1 cup salsa
- 1 cup small tomatoes, diced, canned choose low-sodium
- 2 tbsp. taco seasoning
- 1/2 cup celery, finely diced
- 1/2 cup carrots, shredded
- 3 tbsp. low-fat sour cream

Directions:

1. Add the turkey to your slow cooker. Season it with taco seasoning, then top with salsa and vegetables.
2. Add in 1/2 cup of water. Set to cook on for 15 minutes (internal temperature should be 165°F when done).

3. Shred the turkey with 2 forks, add in sour cream, and stir. Enjoy.

Nutrition:

- Calories: 178 kcal
- Fat: 4 g
- Carbs: 7 g
- Fiber: 2 g
- Protein: 27 g

118. Sriracha Lime Chicken and Apple Salad

Preparation Time: 10 minutes

Cooking Time: 15 minutes

Servings: 4

Ingredients:

Sriracha Lime Chicken:

- 2 organic chicken breasts
- 3 tbsp. sriracha
- 1 lime, juiced
- 1/4 tsp. fine sea salt
- 1/4 tsp. freshly ground pepper

Fruit Salad:

- 4 apples, peeled, cored and diced
- 1 cup organic grape tomatoes
- 1/3 cup red onion, finely chopped

Lime Vinaigrette:

- 1/3 cup light olive oil
- 1/4 cup apple cider vinegar
- 2 limes, juiced
- A fine sea salt dash

Directions:

1. Use salt and pepper to season the chicken on both sides. Spread on the sriracha and lime and let sit for 20 minutes.
2. Cook the chicken per side over medium heat, or until done. Grill the apple with the chicken.
3. Meanwhile, whisk together the dressing and season to taste.
4. Arrange the salad, topping it with red onion and tomatoes.
5. Serve as a side to the chicken and apple.

Nutrition:

- Calories: 484 kcal
- Fat: 28 g
- Carbs: 32 g
- Fiber: 8 g
- Protein: 30 g

119. Pan-Seared Scallops with Lemon-Ginger Vinaigrette

Preparation Time: 10 minutes

Cooking Time: 10 minutes

Servings: 2

Ingredients:

- 1 pound sea scallops
- 1 tbsp. extra-virgin olive oil
- 1/4 tsp. sea salt
- 2 tbsp. lemon-ginger vinaigrette
- A freshly ground black pepper pinch

Directions:

1. Heat the olive oil in a non-stick skillet or pan over medium-high heat until it starts shimmering.
2. Add the scallops to the skillet or pan after seasoning them with pepper and salt. Cook for 3 minutes per side or until the fish is only opaque.
3. Serve with a dollop of vinaigrette on top.

Nutrition:

- Calories: 280 kcal
- Fat: 16
- Carbs: 5 g
- Sugar: 1 g
- Fiber: 0 g

- Protein: 29 g
- Sodium: 508 mg

120. Roasted Salmon and Asparagus

Preparation Time: 5 minutes

Cooking Time: 15 minutes

Servings: 2

Ingredients:

- 1 tbsp. extra-virgin olive oil
- 1 pound salmon, cut into two fillets
- 1/2 lemon zest and slices
- 1/2 pound asparagus spears, trimmed
- 1 tsp. sea salt, divided
- 1/8 tsp. freshly cracked black pepper

Directions:

1. Preheat the oven to 425ºF.
2. Stir the asparagus with half of salt and olive oil. At the base of a roasting tray, spread in a continuous sheet.
3. Season the salmon with salt and pepper. Place the asparagus on top of the skin-side down.
4. Lemon zest should be sprinkled over the asparagus, salmon, and lemon slices. Set them over the top.
5. Roast for around 15 minutes until the flesh of the fish is opaque in the preheated oven.

Nutrition:

- Calories: 308 kcal
- Fat: 18 g
- Carbs: 5 g
- Sugar: 2 g
- Fiber: 2 g
- Protein: 36 g
- Sodium: 542 mg

121. Orange and Maple-Glazed Salmon

Preparation Time: 15 minutes

Cooking Time: 15 minutes

Servings: 2

Ingredients:

- 1 orange zest
- 1 tbsp. low-sodium soy sauce
- 2 (4–6 ounces) salmon fillets, pin bones removed
- 1 orange juice
- 2 tbsp. pure maple syrup
- 1 tsp. garlic powder

Directions:

1. Preheat the oven to 400ºF.
2. Set the orange juice and zest, soy sauce, maple syrup, and garlic powder in a little shallow bowl.
3. Place the salmon parts in the dish flesh-side down. Allow resting 10 minutes for marinating.
4. Put the salmon on a rimmed baking dish, skin-side up, and bake for 15 minutes, or until the flesh is opaque.

Nutrition:

- Calories: 297 kcal
- Fat: 11
- Carbs: 18 g
- Sugar: 15 g
- Fiber: 1 g
- Protein: 34 g
- Sodium: 528 mg

122. Cod with Ginger and Black Beans

Preparation Time: 10 minutes

Cooking Time: 15 minutes

Servings: 2

Ingredients:

- 2 (6 ounces) cod fillets
- 1/2 tsp. sea salt, divided

- 3 minced garlic cloves
- 2 tbsp. chopped fresh cilantro leaves
- 1 tbsp. extra-virgin olive oil
- 1/2 tbsp. grated fresh ginger
- 2 tbsp. freshly ground black pepper
- 1/2 (14 ounces) can black beans, drained

Directions:

1. Heat the olive oil in a big non-stick skillet or pan over medium-high heat until it starts shimmering.
2. Half of the salt, ginger, and pepper are used to season the fish. Cook for around 4 minutes per side in the hot oil until the fish is opaque. Detach the cod from the pan and place it on a plate with aluminum foil tented over it.
3. Add the garlic to the skillet or pan and return it to the heat. Cook for 30 seconds while continuously stirring.
4. Mix the black beans and the remaining salt. Cook, stirring regularly, for 5 minutes.
5. Add the cilantro and serve the black beans on top of the cod.

Nutrition:

- Calories: 419 kcal
- Fat: 2 g
- Carbs: 33 g
- Sugar: 1 g
- Fiber: 8 g
- Protein: 50 g
- Sodium: 605 mg

123. Halibut Curry

Preparation Time: 10 minutes

Cooking Time: 10 minutes

Servings: 2

Ingredients:

- 1 tsp. ground turmeric
- 1 pound halibut, skin, and bones removed, cut into 1-inch pieces
- 1/2 (14 ounces) can coconut milk
- 1/8 tsp. ground black pepper
- 1 tbsp. extra-virgin olive oil
- 1 tsp. curry powder
- 2 cups no-salt-added chicken broth
- 1/4 tsp. sea salt

Directions:

1. Heat the olive oil in a non-stick skillet or pan over medium-high heat until it starts shimmering.
2. Add the curry powder and turmeric to a bowl. To bloom the spices, cook for 2 minutes, stirring continuously.
3. Stir in halibut, coconut milk, chicken broth, pepper, and salt. Lower the heat to medium-low and bring to a simmer. Cook, stirring regularly, for 6–7 minutes, or until the fish is opaque.

Nutrition:

- Calories: 429 kcal
- Fat: 47 g
- Carbs: 5 g
- Sugar: 1 g
- Fiber: 1 g
- Protein: 27 g
- Sodium: 507 mg

124. Chicken Cacciatore

Preparation Time: 10 minutes

Cooking Time: 15 minutes

Servings: 2

Ingredients:

- 1 pound skinless chicken, cut into bite-size pieces
- 1/4 cup black olives, chopped
- 1/2 tsp. onion powder
- A freshly ground black pepper pinch
- 1 tbsp. extra-virgin olive oil
- 1 (28 ounces) can crushed tomatoes, drained
- 1/2 tsp. garlic powder
- 1/4 tsp. sea salt

Directions:

1. Heat the olive oil in a non-stick skillet or pan over medium-high heat until it starts shimmering.
2. Cook until the chicken is browned.
3. Add the tomatoes, garlic powder, olives, salt, onion powder, and pepper, then stir to combine. Cook, stirring regularly, for 10 minutes.

Nutrition:

- Calories: 305 kcal
- Fat: 11 g
- Carbs: 34 g
- Sugar: 23 g
- Fiber: 13 g
- Protein: 19 g
- Sodium: 1.171 mg

125. Chicken and Bell Pepper Saute

Preparation Time: 5 minutes

Cooking Time: 15 minutes

Servings: 2

Ingredients:

- 1 chopped bell pepper
- 1 pound skinless chicken breasts, cut into bite-size pieces
- 1 ½ tbsp. extra-virgin olive oil
- 1/2 chopped onion
- 3 minced garlic cloves
- 1/8 tsp. ground black pepper
- 1/4 tsp. sea salt

Directions:

1. Heat the olive oil in a non-stick skillet or pan over medium-high heat until it starts shimmering.
2. Add the onion, red bell pepper, and chicken. Cook, stirring regularly, for 10 minutes.
3. Stir in the salt, garlic, and pepper in a mixing bowl. Cook for 30 seconds while continuously stirring.

Nutrition:

- Calories: 179 kcal
- Fat: 13 g
- Carbs: 6 g
- Sugar: 3 g
- Fiber: 1 g
- Protein: 10 g
- Sodium: 265 mg

126. Chicken Salad Sandwiches

Preparation Time: 15 minutes

Cooking Time: 0 minutes

Servings: 2

Ingredients:

- 2 tbsp. anti-inflammatory mayonnaise
- 1 tbsp. chopped fresh tarragon leaves
- 1 cup chicken, chopped, cooked, and skinless (from 1 rotisserie chicken)
- 1/2 minced red bell pepper
- 1 tsp. Dijon mustard
- 4 slices whole-wheat bread
- 1/4 tsp. sea salt

Directions:

1. Combine the chicken, red bell pepper, mayonnaise, mustard, tarragon, and salt in a medium mixing bowl.
2. Spread on 2 pieces of bread and top it with the remaining bread.

Nutrition:

- Calories: 315 kcal
- Fat: 9 g
- Carbs: 30 g
- Sugar: 6 g
- Fiber: 4 g
- Protein: 28 g
- Sodium: 677 mg

127. Rosemary Chicken

Preparation Time: 15 minutes

Cooking Time: 15 minutes

Servings: 2

Ingredients:

- 1 tbsp. extra-virgin olive oil
- 1 pound chicken breast tenders
- 1 tbsp. chopped fresh rosemary leaves
- 1/8 tsp. ground black pepper
- 1/4 tsp. sea salt

Directions:

1. Preheat the oven to 425ºF.
2. Set the chicken tenders on a baking sheet with a rim. Sprinkle with salt, rosemary, and pepper after brushing them with olive oil.
3. For 15 minutes, keep in the oven, just before the juices run clear.

Nutrition:

- Calories: 389 kcal
- Fat: 20 g
- Carbs: 1 g
- Sugar: 0 g
- Fiber: 1 g
- Protein: 49 g
- Sodium: 381 mg

128. Gingered Turkey Meatballs

Preparation Time: 10 minutes

Cooking Time: 10 minutes

Servings: 2

Ingredients:

- 1/2 cup shredded cabbage
- 1/2 tbsp. grated fresh ginger
- 1/2 tsp. onion powder
- 1 pound ground turkey
- 2 tbsp. chopped fresh cilantro leaves
- 1/2 tsp. garlic powder
- 1/4 tsp. sea salt
- 1 tbsp. olive oil
- A freshly ground black pepper pinch

Directions:

1. Combine the cabbage, turkey, cilantro, ginger, onion powder, garlic powder, pepper, and salt in a big mixing bowl. Mix well. Make 10 (3/4 inch) meatballs out of the turkey mixture.
2. Heat the oil in a big non-stick skillet or pan over medium-high heat until it starts shimmering.
3. Cook for about 10 minutes, rotating the meatballs while they brown and you are done.

Nutrition:

- Calories: 408 kcal
- Fat: 26 g
- Carbs: 4 g
- Sugar: 1 g
- Fiber: 1 g
- Protein: 47 g
- Sodium: 426 mg

Chapter 7. Recipes With High Fiber

129. Vitamins Packed Green Juice

Preparation Time: 10 minutes

Servings: 2

Ingredients:

- 6 pears, cored and chopped
- 3 celery stalks
- 3 C. fresh kale
- 2 tbsp. fresh parsley

Directions:

1. Place all the ingredients in a blender and pulse until well combined.
2. Through a cheesecloth-lined strainer, strain the juice and transfer into 2 glasses.
3. Serve immediately.

Nutrition:

- Calories: 209 kcal
- Carbs: 50.5 g
- Protein: 5.1 g
- Fat: 0.9 g
- Sugar: 26.2 g
- Sodium: 66 mg
- Fiber: 15.2 g

130. Healthier Breakfast Juice

Preparation Time: 10 minutes

Servings: 2

Ingredients:

- 2 large Granny Smith apples, cored and sliced
- 4 medium carrots, peeled and chopped
- 2 medium grapefruit, peeled and seeded
- 1 C. fresh kale
- 1 tsp. fresh lemon juice

Directions:

1. Place all the ingredients in a blender and pulse until well combined.
2. Through a cheesecloth-lined strainer, strain the juice and transfer into 2 glasses.
3. Serve immediately.

Nutrition:

- Calories: 265 kcal
- Carbs: 67 g
- Protein: 4.2 g
- Fat: 0.7 g
- Sugar: 47.1 g
- Sodium: 101 mg
- Fiber: 11.7 g

131. Summer Perfect Smoothie

Preparation Time: 10 minutes

Servings: 2

Ingredients:

- 2 C. frozen peaches, pitted
- ½ C. rolled oats
- ¼ tsp. ground cinnamon
- 1½ C. plain yogurt
- ½ C. fresh orange Juice

Directions:

1. In a high-speed blender, add all the ingredients and pulse until smooth and creamy.
2. Transfer the smoothie into 2 serving glasses and serve immediately.

Nutrition:

- Calories: 328 kcal
- Carbs: 56 g
- Protein: 15 g
- Fat: 4.1 g
- Sugar: 41 g
- Sodium: 131 mg

- Fiber: 5 g

132. Filling Breakfast Smoothie

Preparation Time: 10 minutes

Servings: 4

Ingredients:

- 2 oz. rolled oats
- 4 apples, peeled, cored, and chopped roughly
- 4 scoops unsweetened vegan protein powder
- 1 tsp. stevia powder
- 1 tsp. ground cinnamon
- 1 tsp. ground nutmeg
- 17 oz. plain yogurt
- 2 C. milk

Directions:

1. In a high-speed blender, add all the ingredients and pulse until smooth and creamy.
2. Transfer the smoothie into 4 serving glasses and serve immediately.

Nutrition:

- Calories: 437 kcal
- Carbs: 55.6 g
- Protein: 38.7 g
- Fat: 6.6 g
- Sugar: 37.5 g
- Sodium: 409 mg
- Fiber: 7.3 g

133. Bright Green Breakfast Bowl

Preparation Time: 10 minutes

Servings: 2

Ingredients:

- 2 C. fresh spinach
- 1 medium avocado, peeled, pitted, and chopped roughly
- 2 scoops unsweetened vegan protein powder
- 3 tbsp. maple syrup
- 2 tbsp. fresh lemon juice
- 1 C. milk
- ¼ C. ice cubes

Directions:

1. In a high-speed blender, place all ingredients and pulse until creamy.
2. Pour into 2 serving bowls and serve immediately with your favorite topping.

Nutrition:

- Calories: 471 kcal
- Carbs: 36.2 g
- Protein: 32.2 g
- Fat: 23.5 g
- Sugar: 24.3 g
- Sodium: 357 mg
- Fiber: 8 g

134. Quickest Breakfast Porridge

Preparation Time: 10 minutes

Cooking Time: 4 minutes

Servings: 4

Ingredients:

- 2 C. milk
- 3 large apples, peeled, cored, and grated
- ½ tsp. vanilla extract
- A ground cinnamon pinch
- 1 banana, peeled and sliced
- ½ small apple, cored and sliced

Directions:

1. In a large pan, add the milk, grated apples, vanilla extract, and cinnamon and mix well.
2. Place the pan over medium-low heat and cook for about 3–4 minutes, stirring occasionally.
3. Transfer the porridge into the serving bowls.

4. Top with the banana and apple slices and serve.

Nutrition:

- Calories: 194 kcal
- Carbs: 40.9 g
- Protein: 5.9 g
- Fat: 3 g
- Sugar: 30 g
- Sodium: 60 mg
- Fiber: 6 g

135. Halloween Morning Oatmeal

Preparation Time: 10 minutes

Cooking Time: 2 minutes

Servings: 2

Ingredients:

- 2 C. hot water
- 1/3 C. pumpkin puree
- 1/3 C. rolled oats
- 1 tsp. ground cinnamon
- 1 tsp. ground ginger
- ¼ tsp. ground nutmeg
- 2 scoops unsweetened vanilla vegan protein powder
- 1 tbsp. maple syrup
- 1 small banana, peeled and sliced

Directions:

1. In a microwave-safe bowl, place water, pumpkin puree, oats, chia seeds, and spices and mix well.
2. Microwave on High for about 2 minutes.
3. Remove the bowl of oatmeal from the microwave and stir in the protein powder and maple syrup.
4. Top with banana slices and serve immediately.

Nutrition:

- Calories: 268 kcal
- Carbs: 34.4 g
- Protein: 28.4 g
- Fat: 2.4 g
- Sugar: 14.8 g
- Sodium: 269 mg
- Fiber: 5 g

136. Authentic Bulgur Porridge

Preparation Time: 10 minutes

Cooking Time: 15 minutes

Servings: 2

Ingredients:

- 2/3 C. milk
- 1/3 C. bulgur, rinsed
- A salt pinch
- 1 ripe banana, peeled and mashed
- 1 large apple, peeled, cored, and chopped

Directions:

1. In a pan, add the soy milk, bulgur, and salt over medium-high heat and bring to a boil.
2. Reduce the heat to low and simmer for about 10 minutes.
3. Remove the pan of bulgur from heat and immediately stir in the mashed banana.
4. Serve warm with the topping of chopped apple.

Nutrition:

- Calories: 231 kcal
- Carbs: 50.6 g
- Protein: 6.5 g
- Fat: 2.4 g
- Sugar: 22.6 g
- Sodium: 121 mg
- Fiber: 8.5 g

137. 2-Grains Porridge

Preparation Time: 10 minutes

Cooking Time: 15 minutes

Servings: 3

Ingredients:

- 2 C. milk
- 2 C. water
- 1 C. old-fashioned oats
- 1/3 C. dried quinoa, rinsed
- 3 tbsp. maple syrup
- ½ tsp. vanilla extract
- 1 large banana, peeled and sliced
- 1 small apple, peeled, cored, and chopped

Directions:

1. In a pan, mix together all the ingredients except for banana and apple over medium heat and bring to a gentle boil.
2. Cook for about 15 minutes, stirring occasionally.
3. Remove from the heat and serve warm with the garnishing of banana and apple.

Nutrition:

- Calories: 384 kcal
- Carbs: 72 g
- Protein: 12.2 g
- Fat: 6.5 g
- Sugar: 32.9 g
- Sodium: 87 mg
- Fiber: 7 g

138. Savory Crepes

Preparation Time: 10 minutes

Cooking Time: 15 minutes

Servings: 4

Ingredients:

- 1¼ C. chickpea flour
- 1½ C. water
- ¼ tsp. red chili powder
- Salt, as required

Directions:

1. In a blender, add all the ingredients and pulse until well combined.
2. Heat a lightly greased nonstick skillet over medium-high heat.
3. Add the desired amount of the mixture and tilt the pan to spread it evenly.
4. Cook for about 3 minutes.
5. Carefully, flip the crepe and cook for about 1–2 minutes.
6. Repeat with the remaining mixture.
7. Serve warm.

Nutrition:

- Calories: 229 kcal
- Carbs: 38.1 g
- Protein: 12.1 g
- Fat: 3.8 g
- Sugar: 6.7 g
- Sodium: 55 mg
- Fiber: 11 g

139. Egg-Free Omelet

Preparation Time: 15 minutes

Cooking Time: 12 minutes

Servings: 4

Ingredients:

- 1 C. chickpea flour
- ¼ tsp. ground turmeric
- ¼ tsp. red chili powder
- A ground cumin pinch
- A sea salt pinch
- 1½-2 C. water
- 1 medium onion, chopped finely
- 2 medium tomatoes, chopped finely
- 2 tbsp. fresh cilantro, chopped
- 2 tbsp. olive oil, divided

Directions:

1. In a large bowl, add the flour, spices, and salt and mix well.
2. Slowly, add the water and mix until well combined.
3. Fold in the onion, tomatoes, and cilantro.
4. In a large non-stick frying pan, heat ½ tbsp. of the oil over medium heat.

5. Add ½ of the tomato mixture and tilt the pan to spread it.
6. Cook for about 5–7 minutes.
7. Place the remaining oil over the "omelet" and carefully flip it over.
8. Cook for about 4–5 minutes or until golden brown.
9. Repeat with the remaining mixture.

Nutrition:

- Calories: 267 kcal
- Carbs: 35.7 g
- Protein: 10.6 g
- Fat: 10.3 g
- Sugar: 8.3 g
- Sodium: 86 mg
- Fiber: 10.2 g

140. Summer Treat Salad

Preparation Time: 15 minutes

Servings: 4

Ingredients:

- 2 large avocados, peeled, pitted, and chopped
- 1 large apple, peeled, pitted, and chopped
- 1 large peach, peeled, pitted, and chopped
- 1 C. cantaloupe, peeled and chopped
- 1 shallot, chopped finely
- 1 seedless cucumber, peeled and chopped
- ¼ C. fresh lime juice
- ¼ C. fresh mint, chopped
- 6 C. lettuce leaves, torn

Directions:

1. In a large salad bowl, add all the ingredients and toss to coat well.
2. Set aside for at least 10–20 minutes before serving.

Nutrition:

- Calories: 262 kcal
- Carbs: 28.7 g
- Protein: 3.7 g
- Fat: 17.1 g
- Sugar: 14.9 g
- Sodium: 20 mg
- Fiber: 9.5 g

141. Secretly Amazing Salad

Preparation Time: 15 minutes

Cooking Time: 15 minutes

Servings: 6

Ingredients:

For Lentils:

- 4 C. water
- 2 C. dried green lentils, rinsed
- 2 large garlic cloves, halved lengthwise
- 2 tbsp. olive oil

For Dressing:

- 1 garlic clove, minced
- ¼ C. fresh lemon juice
- 2 tbsp. olive oil
- 1 tsp. maple syrup
- 1 tsp. Dijon mustard
- Salt and freshly ground black pepper, to taste

For Salad:

- 1½ (15-oz.) cans chickpeas, rinsed and drained
- 2 large avocados, peeled, pitted, and chopped
- 2 C. radishes, trimmed and sliced
- ¼ C. fresh mint leaves, chopped

Directions:

1. For lentils: in a medium pot, add all ingredients over medium-high heat and bring to a boil.
2. Reduce the heat to low and simmer for about 12 minutes or until the lentils are cooked through and tender.
3. Drain the lentils and discard the garlic cloves.

For dressing:

1. Add all ingredients in a small bowl and beat until well combined.
2. In a large serving bowl, add lentils, chickpeas, radishes, avocados, and mint and mix.
3. Add the dressing and toss to coat well.
4. Serve immediately.

Nutrition:

- Calories: 561 kcal
- Carbs: 66.4 g
- Protein: 24.9 g
- Fat: 22.2 g
- Sugar: 3.2 g
- Sodium: 96 mg
- Fiber: 29.2 g

142. Crowd-Pleasing Salad

Preparation Time: 15 minutes

Servings: 5

Ingredients:

- 2 C. cooked quinoa
- 2 C. canned red kidney beans, rinsed and drained
- 5 C. fresh baby spinach
- ¼ C. tomatoes, peeled, seeded, and chopped
- ¼ C. fresh dill, chopped
- ¼ C. fresh parsley, chopped
- 3 tbsp. fresh lemon juice
- Salt and freshly ground black pepper, to taste

Directions:

1. In a large bowl, add all the ingredients and toss to coat well.
2. Serve immediately.

Nutrition:

- Calories: 354 kcal
- Carbs: 62.7 g
- Protein: 16.6 g
- Fat: 4.8 g
- Sugar: 2.5 g
- Sodium: 331 mg
- Fiber: 11.5 g

143. South Western Salad

Preparation Time:15 minutes

Servings: 6

Ingredients:

For Dressing:

- 2 tbsp. fresh lime juice
- 2 tbsp. maple syrup
- 1 tbsp. Dijon mustard
- ½ tsp. ground cumin
- 1 tsp. garlic powder
- Salt and freshly ground black pepper, to taste
- ¼ C. extra-virgin olive oil

For Salad:

- 2 C. fresh mango, peeled, pitted, and cubed
- 2 tbsp. fresh lime juice, divided
- 2 avocados, peeled, pitted, and cubed
- A salt pinch
- 1 C. cooked quinoa
- 2 (14-oz.) cans black beans, rinsed and drained
- 1 small red onion, chopped
- ½ C. fresh cilantro, chopped
- 6 C. romaine lettuce, shredded

Directions:

For dressing:

1. In a blender, add all the ingredients except oil and pulse until well combined.
2. While the motor is running, gradually add the oil and pulse until smooth.

For salad:

1. In a bowl, add the mango and 1 tbsp. of lime juice and toss to coat well.
2. In another bowl, add the avocado, a pinch of salt, and remaining lime juice and toss to coat well.

3. In a large serving bowl, add the mango, avocado, and remaining salad ingredients and mix.
4. Place the dressing and toss to coat well.
5. Serve immediately.

Nutrition:

- Calories: 555 kcal
- Carbs: 71.5 g
- Protein: 18.1 g
- Fat: 24.4 g
- Sugar: 13 g
- Sodium: 69 mg
- Fiber: 19.7 g

144. Great Luncheon Salad

Preparation Time: 20 minutes

Cooking Time: 5 minutes

Servings: 4

Ingredients:

For Salad:

- ½ C. homemade vegetable broth
- ½ C. couscous
- 3 C. canned red kidney beans, rinsed and drained
- 2 large tomatoes, peeled, seeded, and chopped
- 5 C. fresh spinach, torn

For Dressing:

- 1 garlic clove, minced
- 2 tbsp. shallots, minced
- 2 tsp. lemon zest, grated finely
- ¼ C. fresh lemon juice
- 2 tbsp. extra-virgin olive oil
- Salt and freshly ground black pepper, to taste

Directions:

1. In a pan, add the broth over medium heat and bring to a boil.
2. Add the couscous and stir to combine.
3. Cover the pan and immediately remove it from the heat.
4. Set aside, covered for about 5–10 minutes or until all the liquid is absorbed.

For salad:

1. In a large serving bowl, add the couscous and remaining ingredients and stir to combine.

For dressing:

1. In another small bowl, add all the ingredients and beat until well combined.
2. Pour the dressing over the salad and gently toss to coat well.
3. Serve immediately.

Nutrition:

- Calories: 341 kcal
- Carbs: 53.2 g
- Protein: 15.7 g
- Fat: 8.5 g
- Sugar: 6.6 g
- Sodium: 670 mg
- Fiber: 13.5 g

145. Flavors Powerhouse Lunch Meal

Preparation Time: 15 minutes

Servings: 2

Ingredients:

- 1 large avocado
- 1¼ C. cooked chickpeas
- ¼ C. celery stalks, chopped
- 1 scallion (greed part), sliced
- 1 small garlic clove, minced
- 1½ tbsp. fresh lemon juice
- ½ tsp. olive oil
- Salt and freshly ground black pepper, to taste
- 1 tbsp. fresh cilantro, chopped

Directions:

1. Cut the avocado in half and then remove the pit.

2. With a spoon, scoop out the flesh from each avocado half.
3. Then, cut half of the avocado flesh into equal-sized cubes.
4. In a large bowl, add avocado cubes and remaining ingredients except for sunflower seeds and cilantro and toss to coat well.
5. Stuff each avocado half with chickpeas mixture evenly.
6. Serve immediately with the garnishing of cilantro.

Nutrition:

- Calories: 403 kcal
- Carbs: 0 g
- Protein: 9.8 g
- Fat: 22.6 g
- Sugar: 1.1 g
- Sodium: 546 mg
- Fiber: 13.8 g

146. Eye-Catching Sweet Potato Boats

Preparation Time: 20 minutes

Cooking Time: 15 minutes

Servings: 2

Ingredients:

For Sweet Potatoes:

- 1 large sweet potato, halved lengthwise
- ½ tbsp. olive oil
- Salt and freshly ground black pepper, to taste

For Filling:

- ½ tbsp. olive oil
- 1/3 C. canned chickpeas, rinsed and drained
- 1 tsp. curry powder
- 1/8 tsp. garlic powder
- 1/3 C. cooked quinoa
- Salt and freshly ground black pepper, to taste
- 1 tsp. fresh lime juice
- 1 tsp. fresh cilantro, chopped

Directions:

1. Preheat the oven to 375° F.
2. Rub each sweet potato half with oil evenly.
3. Arrange the sweet potato halves onto a baking sheet, cut side down, and sprinkle with salt and black pepper.
4. Bake for about 15 minutes or until sweet potato becomes tender.
5. Meanwhile, for filling: In a skillet, heat the oil over medium heat and cook the chickpeas, curry powder, and garlic powder for about 6–8 minutes, stirring frequently.
6. Stir in the cooked quinoa, salt, and black pepper and remove from the heat.
7. Remove from the oven and arrange each sweet potato halves onto a plate.
8. With a fork, fluff the flesh of each half slightly.
9. Place chickpeas mixture in each half and drizzle with lime juice
10. Serve immediately with the garnishing of cilantro and sesame seeds.

Nutrition:

- Calories: 286 kcal
- Carbs: 43 g
- Protein: 8.2 g
- Fat: 9.7 g
- Sugar: 6.6 g
- Sodium: 175 mg
- Fiber: 8 g

147. Mexican Enchiladas

Preparation Time: 15 minutes

Cooking Time: 15 minutes

Servings: 8

Ingredients:

- 1 (14-oz.) can red beans, drained, rinsed, and mashed
- 2 C. cheddar cheese, grated
- 2 C. tomato sauce

- ½ C. onion, chopped
- ¼ C. black olives, pitted and sliced
- 2 tsp. garlic salt
- 8 whole-wheat tortillas

Directions:

1. Preheat the oven to 350°F.
2. In a medium bowl, add the mashed beans, cheese, 1 C. of tomato sauce, onions, olives, and garlic salt and mix well.
3. Place about 1/3 C. of the bean mixture along the center of each tortilla.
4. Roll up each tortilla and place enchiladas in a large baking dish.
5. Place the remaining tomato sauce on top of the filled tortillas.
6. Bake for about 15 minutes.
7. Serve warm.

Nutrition:

- Calories: 358 kcal
- Carbs: 46.2 g
- Protein: 20.6 g
- Fat: 11.2 g
- Sugar: 4.5 g
- Sodium: 550 mg
- Fiber: 10.3 g

148. Unique Banana Curry

Preparation Time: 15 minutes

Cooking Time: 15 minutes

Servings: 3

Ingredients:

- 2 tbsp. olive oil
- 2 yellow onions, chopped
- 8 garlic cloves, minced
- 2 tbsp. curry powder
- 1 tbsp. ground ginger
- 1 tbsp. ground cumin
- 1 tsp. ground turmeric
- 1 tsp. ground cinnamon
- 1 tsp. red chili powder
- Salt and freshly ground black pepper, to taste
- 2/3 C. plain yogurt
- 1 C. tomato puree
- 2 bananas, peeled and sliced
- 3 tomatoes, peeled, seeded, and chopped finely

Directions:

1. In a large pan, heat the oil over medium heat and sauté onion for about 4–5 minutes.
2. Add the garlic, curry powder, and spices, and sauté for about 1 minute.
3. Add the yogurt and tomato sauce and bring to a gentle boil.
4. Stir in the bananas and simmer for about 3 minutes.
5. Stir in the tomatoes and simmer for about 1–2 minutes.
6. Remove from the heat and serve hot.

Nutrition:

- Calories: 318 kcal
- Carbs: 49.7 g
- Protein: 9 g
- Fat: 12.2 g
- Sugar: 24.2 g
- Sodium: 138 mg
- Fiber: 9.5 g

149. Vegan-Friendly Platter

Preparation Time: 10 minutes

Cooking Time: 15 minutes

Servings: 4

Ingredients:

- 1 tbsp. olive oil
- 2 small onions, chopped
- 5 garlic cloves, chopped finely
- 1 tsp. of dried oregano
- 1 tsp. ground cumin
- ½ tsp. ground ginger
- Salt and freshly ground black pepper, to taste

- 2 cups tomatoes, peeled, seeded, and chopped
- 2 (13½-oz.) cans black beans, rinsed and drained
- ½ C. homemade vegetable broth

Directions:

1. In a pan, heat the olive oil over medium heat and cook the onion for about 5 minutes, stirring frequently.
2. Add the garlic, oregano, spices, salt, and black pepper and cook for about 1 minute.
3. Add the tomatoes and cook for about 1–2 minutes.
4. Add in the beans and broth and bring to a boil.
5. Reduce the heat to medium-low and simmer, covered for about 10 minutes.
6. Serve hot.

Nutrition:

- Calories: 327 kcal
- Carbs: 54.1 g
- Protein: 19.1 g
- Fat: 5.1 g
- Sugar: 4 g
- Sodium: 595 mg
- Fiber: 18.8 g

150. Armenian Style Chickpeas

Preparation Time: 15 minutes
Cooking Time: 15 minutes
Servings: 4
Ingredients:

- 2 tbsp. olive oil
- 1 medium yellow onion, chopped
- 4 garlic cloves, minced
- 1 tsp. dried thyme, crushed
- 1 tsp. dried oregano, crushed
- ½ tsp. paprika
- 1 C. tomato, chopped finely
- 2½ C. canned chickpeas, rinsed and drained
- 5 C. Swiss chards, chopped
- 2 tbsp. water
- 2 tbsp. fresh lemon juice
- Salt and freshly ground black pepper, to taste
- 3 tbsp. fresh basil, chopped

Directions:

1. In a skillet, heat the olive oil over medium heat and sauté the onion for about 6–8 minutes.
2. Add the garlic, herbs, and paprika, and sauté for about 1 minute.
3. Add the Swiss chard and 2 tbsp. water and cook for about 2–3 minutes.
4. Add the tomatoes and chickpeas and cook for about 2–3 minutes.
5. Add in the lemon juice, salt, and black pepper and remove from the heat.
6. Serve hot with the garnishing of basil.

Nutrition:

- Calories: 260 kcal
- Carbs: 34 g
- Protein: 12 g
- Fat: 8.6 g
- Sugar: 3.1 g
- Sodium: 178 mg
- Fiber: 9 g

151. Protein-Packed Soup

Preparation Time: 15 minutes
Cooking Time: 15 minutes
Servings: 8
Ingredients:

- 2 tbsp. olive oil
- 1½ lb. ground turkey
- Salt and freshly ground black pepper, to taste
- 1 large carrot, peeled and chopped
- 1 large celery stalk, chopped
- 1 large onion, chopped

- 6 garlic cloves, chopped
- 1 tsp. dried rosemary
- 1 tsp. dried oregano
- 2 large potatoes, peeled and chopped
- 8–9 C. chicken bone broth
- 4–5 C. tomatoes, peeled, seeded, and chopped
- 2 C. dry lentils
- ¼ C. fresh parsley, chopped

Directions:

1. In a large soup pan, heat the olive oil over medium-high heat and cook the turkey for about 5 minutes or until browned.
2. With a slotted spoon, transfer the turkey into a bowl and set it aside.
3. In the same pan, add the carrot, celery onion, garlic, and dried herbs over medium heat and cook for about 3 minutes.
4. Add the potatoes and cook for about 3 minutes.
5. Add the cooked turkey, tomatoes, and broth and bring to a boil over high heat.
6. Reduce the heat to low and cook, covered for about 5 minutes.
7. Add the lentils and cook, covered for about 5 minutes.
8. Stir in black pepper and remove from the heat.
9. Serve hot with the garnishing of parsley.

Nutrition:

- Calories: 485 kcal
- Carbs: 44.6 g
- Protein: 43 g
- Fat: 16.5 g
- Sugar: 8.5 g
- Sodium: 452 mg
- Fiber: 16.6 g

152. One-Pot Dinner Soup

Preparation Time: 15 minutes

Cooking Time: 15 minutes

Servings: 4

Ingredients:

- 1 tbsp. olive oil
- 1 C. yellow onion, chopped
- ½ C. carrots, peeled and chopped
- ½ C. celery, chopped
- 2 garlic cloves, minced
- 4 C. homemade vegetable broth
- 2½ C. sweet potatoes, peeled and chopped
- 1 C. red lentils, rinsed
- 1½ tbsp. fresh lemon juice
- Salt and freshly ground black pepper, to taste
- 2 tbsp. fresh cilantro, chopped

Directions:

1. In a large Dutch oven, heat the oil over medium heat and sauté the onion, carrot, and celery for about 5–7 minutes.
2. Add the garlic and sauté for about 1 minute.
3. Add the sweet potatoes and cook for about 1–2 minutes.
4. Add in the broth and bring to a boil.
5. Reduce the heat to low and simmer, covered for about 5 minutes.
6. Stir in the red lentils and gain bring to a boil over medium-high heat.
7. Reduce the heat to low and simmer, covered for about 15 minutes or until desired doneness.
8. Stir in the lemon juice, salt, and black pepper and remove from the heat.
9. Serve hot with the garnishing of cilantro.

Nutrition:

- Calories: 471 kcal
- Carbs: 61 g

- Protein: 19.3 g
- Fat: 5.6 g
- Sugar: 4.4 g
- Sodium: 836 mg
- Fiber: 19.7 g

153. 3-Beans Soup

Preparation Time: 15 minutes

Cooking Time: 15 minutes

Servings: 12

Ingredients:

- ¼ C. olive oil
- 1 large onion, chopped
- 1 large sweet potato, peeled and cubed
- 3 carrots, peeled and chopped
- 3 celery stalks, chopped
- 3 garlic cloves, minced
- 2 tsp. dried thyme, crushed
- 1 tbsp. red chili powder
- 1 tbsp. ground cumin
- 4 large tomatoes, peeled, seeded, and chopped finely
- 2 (16-oz.) cans great Northern beans, rinsed and drained
- 2 (15¼-oz.) cans red kidney beans, rinsed and drained
- 1 (15-oz.) can black beans, drained and rinsed
- 12 C. homemade vegetable broth
- 1 C. fresh cilantro, chopped
- Salt and freshly ground black pepper, to taste

Directions:

1. In a Dutch oven, heat the oil over medium heat and sauté the onion, sweet potato, carrot, and celery for about 6–8 minutes.
2. Add the garlic, thyme, chili powder, and cumin and sauté for about 1 minute.
3. Add in the tomatoes and cook for about 2–3 minutes.
4. Add the beans and broth and bring to a boil over medium-high heat.
5. Cover the pan with a lid and cook for about 15 minutes.
6. Stir in the cilantro and remove from heat.
7. Serve hot.

Nutrition:

- Calories: 411 kcal
- Carbs: 69.7 g
- Protein: 22.7 g
- Fat: 5.7 g
- Sugar: 7.1 g
- Sodium: 931 mg
- Fiber: 18.9 g

154. Heavenly Tasty Stew

Preparation Time: 15 minutes

Cooking Time: 15 minutes

Servings: 6

Ingredients:

- ¼ C. olive oil
- 1 large yellow onion, chopped
- 8 oz. fresh shiitake mushrooms, sliced
- 2 large tomatoes, chopped
- 2 tbsp. garlic, chopped finely
- 2 bay leaves
- 2 tbsp. mixed Italian herbs (rosemary, thyme, basil), chopped
- 1 tsp. cayenne pepper
- 4 C. homemade vegetable broth
- 2 tbsp. apple cider vinegar
- 1 C. whole-wheat fusilli pasta
- 1/3 C. nutritional yeast
- 8 oz. fresh collard greens
- 1 (15-oz.) can cannellini beans, drained and rinsed
- Salt and freshly ground black pepper, to taste

Directions:

1. In a large pan, heat the oil over medium heat and sauté the onion, mushrooms, potato, and tomato for about 4–5 minutes.

2. Add the garlic, bay leaves, herbs, and cayenne pepper and sauté for about 1 minute.
3. Add the broth and bring to a boil.
4. Stir in the vinegar, pasta, and nutritional yeast and again bring to a boil.
5. Reduce the heat to medium-low and simmer, covered for about 10 minutes.
6. Uncover and stir in the greens and beans.
7. Simmer for about 4–5 minutes.
8. Stir in the salt and black pepper and remove from the heat.
9. Serve hot.

Nutrition:

- Calories: 314 kcal
- Carbs: 46 g
- Protein: 14.4 g
- Fat: 10 g
- Sugar: 6.2 g
- Sodium: 489 mg
- Fiber: 12.3 g

155. Thanksgiving Dinner Chili

Preparation Time: 15 minutes

Cooking Time: 15 minutes

Servings: 6

Ingredients:

- 2 tbsp. olive oil
- 1 red bell pepper, seeded and chopped
- 1 onion, chopped
- 2 garlic cloves, chopped
- 1 lb. lean ground turkey
- 2 C. water
- 3 C. tomatoes, chopped finely
- 1 tsp. ground cumin
- ½ tsp. ground cinnamon
- 1 (15-oz.) can red kidney beans, rinsed and drained
- 1 (15-oz.) cans black beans, rinsed and drained
- ¼ C. scallion greens, chopped

Directions:

1. In a large Dutch oven, heat the olive oil over medium-low heat and sauté bell pepper, onion, and garlic for about 5 minutes.
2. Add the turkey and cook for about 5–6 minutes, breaking up the chunks with a wooden spoon.
3. Add the water, tomatoes, and spices and bring to a boil over high heat.
4. Reduce the heat to medium-low and stir in beans and corn.
5. Simmer, covered for about 10 minutes, stirring occasionally.
6. Serve hot with the topping of scallion greens.

Nutrition:

- Calories: 366 kcal
- Carbs: 40.6 g
- Protein: 28.7 g
- Fat: 11.2 g
- Sugar: 4.5 g
- Sodium: 100 mg
- Fiber: 13.4 g

156. Meatless Monday Chili

Preparation Time: 15 minutes

Cooking Time: 15 minutes

Servings: 4

Ingredients:

- 2 tbsp. avocado oil
- 1 medium onion, chopped
- 1 carrot, peeled and chopped
- 1 small bell pepper, seeded and chopped
- 1 lb. fresh mushrooms, sliced
- 2 garlic cloves, minced
- 2 tsp. dried oregano
- 1 tbsp. red chili powder
- 1 tbsp. ground cumin

- Salt and freshly ground black pepper, to taste
- 8 oz. canned red kidney beans, rinsed and drained
- 8 oz. canned white kidney beans, rinsed and drained
- 2 C. tomatoes, peeled, seeded, and chopped finely
- 1½ C. homemade vegetable broth

Directions:

1. In a large Dutch oven, heat the oil over medium-low heat and cook the onions, carrot, and bell pepper for about 10 minutes, stirring frequently.
2. Increase the heat to medium-high.
3. Stir in the mushrooms and garlic and cook for about 5–6 minutes, stirring frequently.
4. Add the oregano, spices, salt, and black pepper and cook for about chili 1–2 minutes.
5. Stir in the beans, tomatoes, and broth and bring to a boil.
6. Reduce the heat to low and simmer, covered for about 15 minutes, stirring occasionally.
7. Serve hot.

Nutrition:

- Calories: 346 kcal
- Carbs: 59.9 g
- Protein: 23.4 g
- Fat: 3.7 g
- Sugar: 10.5 g
- Sodium: 545 mg
- Fiber: 16.7 g

157. Beans Trio Chili

Preparation Time: 15 minutes

Cooking Time: 15 minutes

Servings: 6

Ingredients:

- 2 tbsp. olive oil
- 1 green bell pepper, seeded and chopped
- 2 celery stalks, chopped
- 1 scallion, chopped
- 3 garlic cloves, minced
- 1 tsp. dried oregano, crushed
- 1 tbsp. red chili powder
- 2 tsp. ground cumin
- 1 tsp. red pepper flakes, crushed
- 1 tsp. ground turmeric
- 1 tsp. onion powder
- 1 tsp. garlic powder
- Salt and freshly ground black pepper, to taste
- 4½ C. tomatoes, peeled, seeded, and chopped finely
- 4 C. water
- 1 (16-oz.) can red kidney beans, rinsed and drained
- 1 (16-oz.) can cannellini beans, rinsed and drained
- ½ of (16-oz.) can black beans, rinsed and drained

Directions:

1. In a large pan, heat the oil over medium heat and cook the bell peppers, celery, scallion, and garlic for about 8–10 minutes, stirring frequently.
2. Add the oregano, spices, salt, black pepper, tomatoes, and water and bring to a boil.
3. Simmer for about 5 minutes.
4. Stir in the beans and simmer for about 10 minutes.
5. Serve hot.

Nutrition:

- Calories: 342 kcal
- Carbs: 56 g
- Protein: 20.3 g
- Fat: 6.1 g
- Sugar: 6 g
- Sodium: 79 mg
- Fiber: 21.3 g

158. Staple Vegan Curry

Preparation Time: 15 minutes

Cooking Time: 15 minutes

Servings: 6

Ingredients:

- 10 oz. whole-wheat pasta
- 1 tbsp. vegetable oil
- 1 medium white onion, chopped
- 3 garlic cloves, minced
- 1 tsp. dried basil, crushed
- 1 tbsp. curry powder
- ¼ tsp. red pepper flakes, crushed
- 2 lb. ripe tomatoes, peeled, seeded, and chopped
- 4 C. cauliflower, cut into bite-sized pieces
- 1 medium red bell pepper, seeded and sliced thinly
- 1 C. water
- 1 (15-oz.) can chickpeas, drained and rinsed
- 1 C. fresh baby spinach
- ¼ C. fresh parsley, chopped
- Salt, to taste

Directions:

1. In a pan of the salted boiling water, add the pasta and cook for about 6–8 minutes or according to the package's directions.
2. Drain the pasta well and set it aside.
3. Heat the oil in a large cast-iron skillet over medium heat and sauté the onion for about 1–2 minutes.
4. Add the garlic, basil, curry powder, and red pepper flakes and sauté for about 1 minute.
5. Stir in the tomatoes, cauliflower, bell pepper, and water, and bring to a gentle boil.
6. Reduce the heat to medium-low and simmer, covered for about 10 minutes.
7. Stir in the chickpeas and cook for about 5 minutes.
8. Add the spinach and cook for about 3–4 minutes.
9. Stir in the pasta and remove from the heat.
10. Serve hot.

Nutrition:

- Calories: 338 kcal
- Carbs: 58.4 g
- Protein: 15.1 g
- Fat: 5.9 g
- Sugar: 10.9 g
- Sodium: 80 mg
- Fiber: 10.3 g

159. Fragrant Vegetarian Curry

Preparation Time: 15 minutes

Cooking Time: 15 minutes

Servings: 8

Ingredients:

- 8 C. water
- ½ tsp. ground turmeric
- 1 C. brown lentils
- 1 C. red lentils
- 1 tbsp. olive oil
- 1 large white onion, chopped
- 3 garlic cloves, minced
- 2 large tomatoes, peeled, seeded, and chopped
- 1½ tbsp. curry powder
- ¼ tsp. ground cloves
- 2 tsp. ground cumin
- 3 carrots, peeled and chopped
- 3 C. pumpkin, peeled, seeded, and cubed into 1-inch size
- 1 granny smith apple, cored and chopped
- 2 C. fresh spinach, chopped
- Salt and freshly ground black pepper, to taste

Directions:

1. In a large pan, add the water, turmeric, and lentils over high heat and bring to a boil.
2. Reduce the heat to medium-low and simmer, covered for about 15 minutes.
3. Drain the lentils, reserving 2½ C. of the cooking liquid.
4. Meanwhile, in another large pan, heat the oil over medium heat and sauté the onion for about 2–3 minutes.
5. Add in the garlic and sauté for about 1 minute.
6. Add the tomatoes and cook for about 2 minutes.
7. Stir in the curry powder and spices and cook for about 1 minute.
8. Add the carrots, potatoes, pumpkin, cooked lentils, and reserved cooking liquid and bring to a gentle boil.
9. Reduce the heat to medium-low and simmer, covered for about 10 minutes or until the desired doneness of the vegetables.
10. Stir in the apple and spinach and simmer for about 3 minutes.
11. Stir in the salt and black pepper and remove from the heat.
12. Serve hot.

Nutrition:

- Calories: 263 kcal
- Carbs: 47 g
- Protein: 14.7 g
- Fat: 2.9 g
- Sugar: 9.7 g
- Sodium: 53 mg
- Fiber: 20 g

160. Omega-3 Rich Dinner Meal

Preparation Time: 15 minutes
Cooking Time: 15 minutes
Servings: 4
Ingredients:

For Lentils:

- ½ lb. French green lentils
- 2 tbsp. extra-virgin olive oil
- 2 C. yellow onions, chopped
- 2 C. scallions, chopped
- 1 tsp. fresh parsley, chopped
- Salt and freshly ground black pepper, to taste
- 1 tbsp. garlic, minced
- 1½ C. carrots, peeled and chopped
- 1½ C. celery stalks, chopped
- 1 large tomato, peeled, seeded, and crushed finely
- 1½ C. chicken bone broth
- 2 tbsp. balsamic vinegar

For Salmon:

1. 2 (8-oz.) skinless salmon fillets
2. 2 tbsp. extra-virgin olive oil
3. Salt and freshly ground black pepper, to taste

Directions:

1. In a heat-proof bowl, soak the lentils in boiling water for 15 minutes.
2. Drain the lentils completely.
3. In a Dutch oven, heat the oil over medium heat and cook the onions, scallions, parsley, salt, and black pepper for about 10 minutes, stirring frequently.
4. Add the garlic and cook for about 2 more minutes.
5. Add the drained lentils, carrots, celery, crushed tomato, and broth and bring to a boil.
6. Reduce the heat to low and simmer, covered for about 10 minutes.
7. Stir in the vinegar, salt, and black pepper and remove from the heat.
8. Meanwhile, for salmon: preheat your oven to 450°F.
9. Rub the salmon fillets with oil and then season with salt and black pepper generously.

10. Heat an oven-proof sauté pan over medium heat and cook the salmon fillets for about 2 minutes, without stirring.
11. Flip the fillets and immediately transfer the pan into the oven.
12. Bake for about 5 minutes or until the desired doneness of salmon.
13. Remove from the oven and place the salmon fillets onto a cutting board.
14. Cut each fillet into 2 portions.
15. Divide the lentil mixture onto serving plates and top each with 1 salmon fillet.
16. Serve hot.

Nutrition:

- Calories: 707 kcal
- Carbs: 50.2 g
- Protein: 16.1 g
- Fat: 29.8 g
- Sugar: 7.9 g
- Sodium: 496 mg
- Fiber: 16.2 g

161. Weekend Dinner Casserole

Preparation Time: 20 minutes

Cooking Time: 15 minutes

Servings: 6

Ingredients:

- 2½ C. water, divided
- 1 C. red lentils
- ½ C. wild rice
- 1 tsp. olive oil
- 1 small onion, chopped
- 3 garlic cloves, minced
- 1/3 C. zucchini, peeled, seeded, and chopped
- 1/3 C. carrot, peeled and chopped
- 1/3 C. celery stalk, chopped
- 1 large tomato, peeled, seeded, and chopped
- 8 oz. tomato sauce
- 1 tsp. ground cumin
- 1 tsp. dried oregano, crushed
- 1 tsp. dried basil, crushed
- Salt and freshly ground black pepper, to taste

Directions:

1. In a pan, add 1 C. of the water and rice over medium-high heat and bring to a rolling boil.
2. Reduce the heat to low and simmer, covered for about 10 minutes.
3. Meanwhile, in another pan, add the remaining water and lentils over medium heat and bring to a rolling boil.
4. Reduce the heat to low and simmer, covered for about 15 minutes.
5. Transfer the cooked rice and lentils into a casserole dish and set aside.
6. Preheat your oven to 350°F.
7. Heat the oil in a large skillet over medium heat and sauté the onion and garlic for about 4-5 minutes.
8. Add the zucchini, carrot, celery, tomato, and tomato paste and cook for about 4–5 minutes.
9. Stir in the cumin, herbs, salt, and black pepper and remove from the heat.
10. Transfer the vegetable mixture into the casserole dish with rice and lentils and stir to combine.
11. Bake for about 15 minutes.
12. Remove from the heat and set aside for about 5 minutes.
13. Cut into equal-sized 6 pieces and serve.

Nutrition:

- Calories: 192 kcal
- Carbs: 34.5 g
- Protein: 11.3 g
- Fat: 1.5 g
- Sugar: 3.9 g
- Sodium: 239 mg
- Fiber: 12 g

162. Family Dinner Pilaf

Preparation Time: 15 minutes

Cooking Time: 15 minutes

Servings: 4

Ingredients:

- 2 tbsp. olive oil
- 2 garlic cloves, minced
- 2 C. fresh mushrooms, sliced
- 1¼ C. brown rice, rinsed
- 2 C. homemade vegetable broth
- Salt and freshly ground black pepper, to taste
- 1 red bell pepper, seeded and chopped
- 4 scallions, chopped
- 1 (16-oz.) can red kidney beans, drained and rinsed
- 2 tbsp. fresh parsley, chopped

Directions:

1. In a large pan, heat the oil over medium heat and sauté the onion for about 4–5 minutes.
2. Add the garlic and mushrooms and cook for about 5–6 minutes.
3. Stir in the rice and cook for about 1–2 minutes, stirring continuously.
4. Stir in the broth, salt, and black pepper and bring to a boil.
5. Reduce the heat to low and simmer, covered for about 15 minutes, stirring occasionally.
6. Add in the bell pepper and beans and cook for about 5–10 minutes or until all the liquid is absorbed. Serve hot with the garnishing of parsley.

Nutrition:

- Calories: 463 kcal
- Carbs: 76.7 g
- Protein: 18.5 g
- Fat: 10.1 g
- Sugar: 3.2 g
- Sodium: 431 mg
- Fiber: 11.6 g

163. Meat-Free Bolognese Pasta

Preparation Time: 20 minutes

Cooking Time: 15 minutes

Servings: 5

Ingredients:

For Bolognese Sauce:

- 5 tbsp. olive oil, divided
- 3 celery stalks, chopped finely
- 1 medium carrot, peeled and chopped finely
- 1 medium onion, chopped finely
- 1 C. quinoa, rinsed
- 3 C. fresh mushrooms, chopped
- 4 garlic cloves, chopped
- ¾ tsp. dried oregano
- ½ tsp. dried thyme
- ¼ tsp. dried rosemary
- ¼ tsp. dried sage
- 1/8 tsp. red pepper flakes
- 1½ C. homemade vegetable broth
- 2 cups tomatoes, peeled, seeded, and crushed finely
- ½-1 C. water
- 1 tbsp. balsamic vinegar
- 4 bay leaves
- 2 tbsp. nutritional yeast
- ¼ C. oat milk
- Salt and freshly ground black pepper, to taste
- ¼ C. fresh basil leaves

For Pasta:

- ¾ lb. whole-wheat pasta (of your choice)

Directions:

1. Preheat your oven to 300°F.
2. In a large Dutch oven, heat 3 tbsp. of the olive oil over medium heat and cook the celery, carrots, and onion for about 10 minutes, stirring frequently.
3. Stir in the quinoa and cook for about 3 minutes.

4. Add the remaining oil and mushrooms and stir to combine.
5. Increase the heat to medium-high and cook for about 5 minutes.
6. Add the garlic, dried herbs, and red pepper flakes and cook for about 1–2 minutes.
7. Add the broth and cook for about 5 minutes.
8. Add the tomatoes, water, vinegar, and bay leaves and bring to a boil.
9. Remove the Dutch oven from heat and transfer it into the oven.
10. Bake, uncovered for about 1½ hours, stirring once after 1 hour.
11. Meanwhile, in a pan of lightly salted boiling water, cook the pasta for about 8–10 minutes or according to the package's instructions.
12. Drin the pasta well.
13. Remove the Dutch oven from the oven and stir in the nutritional yeast and oat milk.
14. Divide the pasta onto serving plates and top with Bolognese sauce.
15. Garnish with basil leaves and serve.

Nutrition:

- Calories: 510 kcal
- Carbs: 71 g
- Protein: 17.1 g
- Fat: 18.3 g
- Sugar: 5.9 g
- Sodium: 241 mg
- Fiber: 6.5 g

164. High-Fiber Dumplings

Preparation Time: 10 minutes

Cooking Time: 10 minutes

Servings: 8

Ingredients:

- 200 g cream quark
- 60 g psyllium husks
- 10 g bamboo fibers
- 1 bowl vegetable broth
- 2 eggs

Directions:

1. Take a bowl and add the psyllium husks along with the bamboo fibers. Mix well with a spoon.
2. Put the eggs in the same bowl, add the cream curd and vegetable stock. Knead well, it's best done by hand. Alternatively, the kneading hooks of the mixer can be used.
3. Set a large saucepan with water and bring to a boil on the stove. In the meantime, moisten your hands with water and roll the dough into 12 balls.
4. Put the balls in hot water and cook for 10 minutes, then serve. High-fiber vegetables like beans and matching sauces also taste great.

Nutrition:

- Calories: 75 kcal
- Carbs: 0.1 g
- Protein: 13.4 g
- Fat: 1.7 g
- Sugar: 0 g
- Sodium: 253 mg

165. Pizza Made with Bamboo Fibers

Preparation Time: 10 minutes

Cooking Time: 15 minutes

Servings: 4

Ingredients:

- 2 eggs
- 60 g bamboo fibers
- 80 g sour cream
- 40 g olive oil
- 150 g grated Gouda cheese
- Salt and pepper

Directions:

1. First, preheat the oven to 180ºC and cover a baking sheet with baking paper.
2. Take a bowl and beat in the eggs. Whisk briefly with a fork, then add the remaining ingredients and knead everything well. This is best done by hand, but you can also work with the dough hook on the mixer.
3. Finally, flavor with salt and pepper to taste, then place the dough on the baking tray and roll out evenly. If necessary, flour the dough with a little bamboo fiber to not stick to the rolling pin.
4. Bake the tray for 10 minutes on the lower rack. The pizza base can now be topped with delicious low-carb foods, depending on your taste. Then bake for another 10 minutes on the lower rack and then enjoy hot.

Nutrition:

- Calories: 599 kcal
- Fat: 19 g
- Carbs: 9 g
- Sugar: 4 g
- Fiber: 2 g
- Protein: 97 g
- Sodium: 520 mg

166. Vegetarian Hamburgers

Preparation Time: 10 minutes

Cooking Time: 15 minutes

Servings: 4

Ingredients:

- 90 g protein flour
- 120 ml egg white
- 100 g carrots, grated
- 2 tbsp. coconut oil
- 100 g low-fat quark
- 2 eggs
- 6 g baking powder
- 20 g gold linseed (alternatively other nuts and grains)
- Preferred spices (Worcester sauce, soy sauce, salt, or chili)
- Preferred topping (tomatoes, cucumbers, radishes, ...)

Directions:

1. First, preheat the oven to 180ºC and line 6–7 muffin tins with paper cases.
2. Take a bowl, add 50 g of flour along with the egg white and carrots, and then stir well. Divide the dough into 6–7 parts and shape a meatball from each one.
3. Now, put 2 tbsp. of coconut oil in a non-stick pan and heat over medium heat until it has melted. Put the meatballs in the hot pan and fry vigorously on both sides.
4. Take a separate bowl, add the remaining flour along with the low-fat quark, eggs, baking powder, and gold linseed.
5. Mix well, then pour into the prepared muffin cups. Bake in the oven for 12 minutes, let the finished rolls cool down well. Finally, cut the rolls in half with a sharp knife, top with a meatball of your choice, and season. Then, skewer the finished burger with a toothpick and enjoy.

Nutrition:

- Calories: 178 kcal
- Fat: 4 g
- Carbs: 7 g
- Fiber: 2 g
- Protein: 27 g

167. Pork Steaks with Avocado

Preparation Time: 10 minutes

Cooking Time: 15 minutes

Servings: 8

Ingredients:

For the salsa:

- 6 limes
- 3 tbsp. fruity olive oil
- 1 ½ dried chili pepper
- Salt and freshly ground pepper
- 2 mangoes (ripe, but still firm)
- 2 shallots
- 2 avocados
- Coriander bunch

For the steaks:

- 4 pork neck steaks (approximately 150 g each)
- 1 tsp. ground anise
- 1 tsp. ground cumin
- Salt
- freshly ground pepper
- 2 tbsp. clarified butter

Directions:

For the salsa:

1. Halve the limes and squeeze them thoroughly, measure out 10 tbsp. of lime juice. Place in a small bowl.
2. Add olive oil and stir well with a whisker. Crumble the chili pepper and mix it into the dressing together with salt and pepper.
3. Now, peel the mangoes with a vegetable peeler, remove the stone and dice the pulp. Finely chop the shallots with a sharp knife.
4. Take a separate bowl, add the mangoes and shallots; stir well.
5. Remove the stone and skin from the avocados, dice the meat and then fill the mango mixture. Immediately, pour the dressing over it so that the avocado doesn't tarnish. Mix gently.
6. Finally, wash the coriander thoroughly under running water and dry it carefully. Remove the tender leaves and also add to the salsa. Mix again.

For the steaks:

1. Preheat the oven to 60ºC. Rinse the steaks under running water and dry them carefully with a little kitchen roll. Sprinkle the anise, cumin, salt, and pepper over them. Place the clarified butter in a pan and heat over medium heat until melted. Set the steaks in the hot pan and fry briefly while turning for 3 minutes.
2. Put the steaks on a piece of aluminum foil and seal it tightly around the steak. Place in the oven and let rest briefly for 3 minutes.
3. Arrange on a plate with the meat juice and salsa. Enjoy immediately!

Nutrition:

- Calories: 303 kcal
- Fat: 14 g
- Carbs: 15 g
- Sugar: 10 g
- Fiber: 2 g
- Protein: 30 g
- Sodium: 387 mg

168. Chicken with Asparagus Salad

Preparation Time: 10 minutes

Cooking Time: 15 minutes

Servings: 4

Ingredients:

- 800 g green asparagus
- 1/2 bunch spring onions
- 3 tbsp. white wine vinegar
- Salt
- Pepper

- 1 tsp. mustard
- 1/2 tsp. honey
- 8 tbsp. olive oil
- 4 chicken breast fillets (approximately 200 g each)
- 250 g sliced breakfast bacon
- 2 tbsp. clarified butter
- Basil leaves for garnishing

Directions:

1. First, preheat the oven to 180ºC and place baking paper on a baking sheet.
2. Take the asparagus and peel only the bottom stick.
3. Remove the woody ends, then wash thoroughly. Halve the asparagus lengthways and cut so that oblique pieces are created. Now, wash the spring onions and cut them into large pieces.
4. Take a bowl, pour the white wine vinegar into it. Also, attach 2 tbsp. of water along with mustard, honey, salt, and pepper. Stir well.
5. Finally, slowly add 6 tbsp. of olive oil, spoon by spoon. Stir.
6. Take the meat, rinse under running water, and dry with a little kitchen roll, then season with salt and pepper on both sides.
7. Take the bacon slices and wrap the meat in them.
8. Put the clarified butter in a non-stick pan and heat over medium fire until the fat has melted. Set the chicken breasts in the hot pan, first placing them to the point where the ends of the bacon slice meet. Turn after 2 minutes and fry again briefly for 2 minutes.
9. Remove from the pan and place on the tray so that the meat can cook in the oven for another 10 minutes.
10. In the meantime, set the remaining olive oil in a pan and heat over medium fire. Put the vegetables in the hot oil and fry briefly. Meanwhile, salt and pepper. After 4 minutes, take the vegetables out of the pan and add them to the vinegar mixture, mix well.
11. Finally, arrange the meat with the asparagus salad on a plate and enjoy immediately.

Nutrition:

- Calories: 256kcal
- Fat: 11 g
- Carbs: 17 g
- Sugar: 8 g
- Fiber: 4 g
- Protein: 45 g
- Sodium: 302 mg

169. Hot Pepper and Lamb Salmon

Preparation Time: 10 minutes

Cooking Time: 15 minutes

Servings: 6

Ingredients:

For the Meat:

- 700 g lamb salmon
- 2 garlic cloves
- 1/2 bunch mint
- 2 sprigs rosemary
- 1/2 bunch oregano
- 10 peppercorns
- 4 tbsp. olive oil
- Salt
- Pepper

For the Peperonata:

- 1 small zucchini
- 2 red peppers
- 2 yellow peppers
- 1 onion
- 3 garlic cloves
- 3 tomatoes
- 1 chili pepper
- 3 tbsp. small capers

- 2 tbsp. olive oil
- Salt
- Pepper
- 2 tbsp. chopped parsley

Directions:

For the Meat:

1. First, rinse the meat under running water and dry it with a little kitchen roll, then carefully remove the tendons and fat. Peel and cut the garlic to make fine slices.
2. Wash the rosemary, oregano, and mint, pat dry carefully. Then, chop the leaves and needles (not too fine). Put the peppercorns in the mortar and press lightly.
3. Take a bowl, add the herbs and peppercorns.
4. Attach 2 tbsp. of olive oil and stir well, then rub the meat with the mixture. Finally, wrap it in foil and refrigerate for 4 hours.
5. Preheat the oven to 70ºC, placing a baking dish in it that will be used for the meat later.
6. Now, take the meat and remove the marinade with the back of a knife, then season with salt and pepper.
7. Set the remaining oil in a pan and heat over medium fire.
8. Place the meat in the hot oil and fry briefly while turning for 2 minutes. Put it in the pan into the oven and cook for another 15 minutes.

For the Peperonata:

1. Wash the zucchini thoroughly and dice it with the skin. Halve and core the peppers, wash them too. Cut so that narrow strips are created. First, peel the onion and garlic, then process into fine cubes.
2. Score the tomatoes, pour hot water, at that time, peel them and remove the seeds. Cut the pulp into small pieces. Alternatively, canned tomatoes can also be used here. Halve and core the chili pepper, wash it well, and cut it into small pieces. Finally, rinse the capers in a sieve and let them drain.
3. Now, pour olive oil over the pan and heat over medium fire. Put the onion in the hot oil and fry briefly, then add the peppers, zucchini, garlic, and chili.
4. Cook for 5 minutes, stirring evenly. Attach tomatoes and season with salt and pepper.
5. Let everything fry for 10 minutes, stir in the capers and cook for another 5 minutes.

Nutrition:

- Calories: 599 kcal
- Fat: 19 g
- Carbs: 9 g
- Sugar: 4 g
- Fiber: 2 g
- Protein: 97 g
- Sodium: 520 mg

170. Pork Rolls À La Ratatouille

Preparation Time: 10 minutes

Cooking Time: 15 minutes

Servings: 8

Ingredients:

For the Ratatouille:

- 2 yellow peppers
- 2 red peppers
- 2 small zucchinis
- 2 red onions
- 3 garlic cloves
- 250 g cherry tomatoes
- A thyme bunch
- 3 tbsp. olive oil
- Salt
- Freshly ground pepper
- 250 ml vegetable stock

- 3 tbsp. tomato paste

For the Pork Rolls:

- 2 basil bunches
- 30 g Parmesan cheese
- 30 g pine nuts
- 5 tbsp. olive oil
- Salt
- Freshly ground pepper
- 75 g sun-dried tomatoes in oil
- 8 small pork schnitzel (approximately 75 g each)

Directions:

For the Ratatouille:

1. First, preheat the oven to 180ºC.
2. Halve and core the peppers, wash thoroughly, and cut so that narrow strips are formed.
3. Wash the zucchini as well, then cut into cubes with the skin on. First, peel the onion and garlic, then cut into strips. Clean the tomatoes thoroughly, cut them in half.
4. Rinse the thyme under running water and pat dry carefully, remove the leaves. Take a bowl, add the vegetables with the thyme and mix well.
5. Flavor with salt, pepper, and olive oil; mix again. Take the frying pan from the oven and distribute the vegetable mixture in it. Bake for 12 minutes.

For the Pork Rolls:

1. Now, rinse the basil with water and shake dry, pluck the leaves and chop finely. Coarsely or finely grate the Parmesan with the grater to taste.
2. Take a small pan, add the pine nuts and briefly toast them without adding any further fat, then put them in the blender. Also, add half of the chopped basil along with the Parmesan and 3 tbsp. of olive oil. Puree everything into a pesto, then season with salt and pepper.
3. Wash the tomatoes and cut them to make strips. Clean the pork as well, dry it with a little kitchen roll and then plate with a meat tenderizer or a saucepan. Sprinkle with salt and pepper, spread some pesto on top.
4. Spread the sun-dried tomatoes and the remaining basil on top, roll into roulades, and set. Add the remaining oil to a pan and heat over medium fire; place the rolls in the hot oil and fry on all sides for 5 minutes.
5. Take a small bowl, add the vegetable stock and tomato paste. Stir.
6. Add the cherry tomatoes and the mixture to the cooked vegetables in the oven. Put the meat on it and bake for another 15 minutes. Enjoy served on a plate with the remaining pesto.

Nutrition:

- Calories: 280 kcal
- Fat: 16
- Carbs: 5 g
- Sugar: 1 g
- Fiber: 0 g
- Protein: 29 g

171. Pepper Fillet with Leek

Preparation Time: 10 minutes

Cooking Time: 15 minutes

Servings: 8

Ingredients:

For the Vegetables:

- 50 g sun-dried tomatoes
- 100 g pine nuts
- 4 large leeks
- 2 tbsp. raisins
- 2 cups Peppercorns
- 2 tbsp. olive oil
- Salt
- Freshly ground pepper

For the Meat:

- 2 tbsp. black pepper

- 4 tbsp. sesame seeds
- 1 tsp. salt
- 4 sprigs rosemary
- 4 beef fillet steaks (approximately 180 g each)
- 4 tbsp. sunflower oil

Directions:

1. Place the tomatoes in a heat-resistant bowl and pour boiling water over them. Let stand for 10 minutes, then take out the tomatoes and chop with a sharp knife.
2. Now, put the pine nuts in a small pan and briefly toast them without adding any further fat, stirring well. Set aside and wash the leek thoroughly and cut so that rings are formed. Rinse the raisins under cold running water.
3. Take a non-stick pan and pour in olive oil. Heat on high and add the leek. Saute briefly, add tomatoes and raisins over low heat and stir well. Cook for 10 minutes, season with salt and pepper. Add the pine nuts, then carefully stir in.
4. At the same time, put the peppercorns in the mortar and coarsely crush them, stir in a small bowl with salt and sesame seeds.
5. Rinse off the rosemary and steaks, then dry them with a little paper towel. Place the steaks with the edges in the pepper mixture so that the spices stick to the edges.
6. Now, heat oil in a non-stick pan on a high level and sear the meat on both sides for 3 minutes. Immediately, wrap in a piece of aluminum foil, covering a sprig of rosemary with it.
7. After resting for 5 minutes, remove the steaks and arrange them on a plate with the leek vegetables. Garnish with meat juice and enjoy instantly.

Nutrition:

- Calories: 504 kcal
- Fat: 39 g
- Carbs: 10 g
- Sugar: 1 g
- Fiber: 2 g
- Protein: 28 g
- Sodium: 755 mg

172. Lamb Chops with Beans

Preparation Time: 10 minutes

Cooking Time: 15 minutes

Servings: 8

Ingredients:

- 1 kg lamb chops
- 2 lemons juice
- Salt
- Pepper
- 150 ml olive oil (approximately)
- 6 garlic cloves
- 6 sprigs rosemary
- 6 sprigs thyme
- 2 onions
- 12 cocktail tomatoes
- 300 g green beans
- 2 shallots
- 70 g bacon
- 2 tsp. butter
- Savory to taste

Directions:

1. First, rinse the lamb chops briefly under running water and carefully dry them with a little kitchen roll. Pour the lemon juice into a small bowl, add 100 ml of olive oil, salt, and pepper; stir well. Take the garlic and remove the peel. Cut so that thin slices are formed, also add to the lemon marinade.
2. Now, put the marinade together with the chops in a freezer bag, squeeze out the air, and seal.
3. Set aside for at least 2 hours and let it soak in.

4. Preheat the oven to 180ºC. Rinse the rosemary, thyme, and pat dry. Take a baking dish and grease it with olive oil. Spread the herb sprigs in it.
5. Add the onions and cut into 4 parts, place them in the mold as well. Wash the tomatoes thoroughly and cut in half depending on the size, then add to the onions.
6. Set the meat out of the marinade and place it on top of the vegetables. Spread the soak and a little olive oil on top. Bake on the middle rack for 15 minutes.
7. In the meantime, take the beans and cut the ends, then wash. Set the water to a boil in a saucepan, season with salt, and add the beans. Cook for 8 minutes. Meanwhile, take the shallots and remove the skin, cut into small cubes. Finely dice the bacon as well.
8. Put the butter in a pan and heat over medium fire until it has melted.
9. Place the shallots and bacon in the hot oil and fry until everything takes on a brown color.
10. Add the beans with a little savory, stir well.
11. Salt and pepper, then serve with the lamb and the bed of vegetables. Enjoy hot.

Nutrition:

- Calories: 413 kcal
- Fat: 20 g
- Carbs: 7 g
- Sugar: 1 g
- Fiber: 1 g
- Protein: 50 g
- Sodium: 358 mg

173. Fillet of Beef on Spring Vegetables

Preparation Time: 10 minutes

Cooking Time: 15 minutes

Servings: 8

Ingredients:

- 500 g green asparagus
- 2 bulbs kohlrabi
- 1 bunch flat-leaf parsley
- 1 bunch tarragon
- Salt
- Pepper
- 4 beef fillet steaks (approximately 150 g each)
- 4 tbsp. olive oil
- 300 ml cream

Directions:

1. Wash the asparagus, peel only the bottom stick with the vegetable peeler. Divide off the woody ends, then cut the asparagus in half. Now, peel the kohlrabi with the knife, cut so that narrow sticks are formed.
2. Rinse the herbs under running water, dry them carefully and remove the leaves. Finely chop with a sharp knife. Take a bowl, pour in 2/3 of the herbs, set aside the rest for now.
3. After that, add the vegetables to the herbs in the bowl, season with salt and pepper, and mix well. Put the mixture in a roasting tube (must be closed on one side).
4. Take a large saucepan, pour water up to 1/3 full. Set on the stove and bring to a boil.
5. In the meantime, rinse the steaks with water and dry them carefully with a little kitchen roll.
6. Season with salt and pepper on both sides. Put the oil in a pan and heat over medium fire.
7. Set the meat in the hot oil and fry briefly on all sides for 3 minutes. Place it on the vegetables in the roasting tube.
8. Pour the oil out of the pan and add in the cream. Bring to the boil briefly so that the roasting loosens, then pour over the meat in the roasting tube.

9. Now, close the hose and add it to the boiling water. Cook gently over low heat and cover for 12 minutes.
10. Finally, arrange the meat with the bed of vegetables on a plate and garnish with the remaining herbs.

Nutrition:

- Calories: 209 kcal
- Fat: 10 g
- Carbs: 21 g
- Sugar: 13 g
- Fiber: 8 g
- Protein: 11 g
- Sodium: 644 mg

174. Bolognese with Zucchini Noodles

Preparation Time: 10 minutes

Cooking Time: 15 minutes

Servings: 4–8

Ingredients:

- 4 zucchini (approximately 200 g each)
- Salt
- 1 onion
- 3 garlic cloves
- 2 tbsp. coconut oil
- 4 tbsp. tomato paste
- 3 tbsp. balsamic vinegar
- 600 g chunky tomatoes (canned)
- 4 sprigs rosemary
- 1 handful basil leaves
- ½ tbsp. Dried oregano
- 1/4 tsp. Dried thyme
- Freshly ground black pepper
- 600 g mixed minced meat
- 2 tbsp. olive oil

Directions:

1. First, wash the zucchini and cut them into thin, narrow slices.
2. For preparing the Bolognese, peel the onion and garlic; cut into fine cubes. Set the oil in a saucepan and heat over medium fire. Put the onion in the hot oil and fry until it becomes translucent.
3. Stir well and fry briefly before adding the tomato paste. Cook them together again, pour in the balsamic vinegar until the bottom can no longer be seen. Bring to a boil, add the tomatoes.
4. Wash the rosemary, and basil then dry them carefully. Pluck the needles and leaves, chop and add to the Bolognese. Season with the remaining herbs to taste.
5. Reduce the heat and simmer gently for 10 minutes before stirring in the minced meat. Cook for another 15 minutes, then cook over high heat for 5 minutes.
6. At the same time, attach olive oil to the zucchini noodles and mix well.
7. Put the oiled zucchini in a pan and cook only briefly over medium heat without becoming too soft.
8. Arrange with the Bolognese on a plate and enjoy hot.

Nutrition:

- Calories: 75 kcal
- Carbs: 0.1 g
- Protein: 13.4 g
- Fat: 1.7 g
- Sugar: 0 g
- Sodium: 253 mg

175. Chicken with Chickpeas

Preparation Time: 10 minutes

Cooking Time: 15 minutes

Servings: 4

Ingredients:

- 12 sun-dried tomatoes in oil
- 2 garlic cloves
- 2 zucchinis
- 500 g chickpeas (canned, drained weight)

- 4 tbsp. olive oil
- 100 ml poultry stock
- 2 bags saffron threads
- Salt
- Freshly ground black pepper
- 1/4 tsp. ground coriander
- 4 chicken breasts (approximately 200 g each)
- 1 tbsp. Ras el Hanout

Directions:

1. First, get the sun-dried tomatoes out of the oil and dry them with a little kitchen roll, then cut them so that narrow strips are formed.
2. Take the garlic, remove the skin and cut it into slices.
3. Wash the zucchini and cut into cubes with the skin on.
4. Rinse the chickpeas in a colander and drain well.
5. Set a saucepan, add 2 tbsp. of olive oil. Warmth on medium heat, add the tomatoes with garlic to the hot oil. Fry briefly for 1 minute.
6. Place the zucchini with chickpeas, stir well and fry briefly together before deglazing with the broth. Add saffron threads, coriander, salt, and pepper. Bring to a boil.
7. Set the heat, cover the saucepan and let the vegetables simmer for 5 minutes.
8. In the meantime, rinse the meat under running water and dry it with a little kitchen roll. Set the remaining oil in a pan and heat over medium fire.
9. For now, sprinkle the meat on both sides with salt, pepper, and Ras el Hanout, then add to the hot oil and fry for 7 minutes, turning.
10. Serve the meat with the vegetables on a large plate and enjoy hot.

Nutrition:

- Calories: 329 kcal
- Fat: 17 g
- Carbs: 9 g
- Sugar: 3 g
- Fiber: 5 g
- Protein: 37 g
- Sodium: 430 mg

176. Ham with Chicory

Preparation Time: 10 minutes

Cooking Time: 15 minutes

Servings: 4–8

Ingredients:

- 4 sprigs chicory (approximately 200 g each)
- 150 g Emmental cheese
- 8 sage leaves
- 40 g butter
- 3 tbsp. orange juice
- Salt
- Pepper
- 8 slices Black Forest ham

Directions:

1. First, preheat the oven to 200ºC.
2. Wash and clean the chicory and cut it lengthways in half. Remove the stalk with a knife.
3. Shred the cheese coarsely or finely with a grater to taste.
4. Rinse the sage leaves under running water and gently shake dry.
5. Put the butter in a pan and heat over medium fire. Extinguish with orange juice and so froth the butter. Add the sage.
6. Place the chicory with the cut side in the hot oil. Reduce the heat and fry for 5 minutes.
7. Remove the chicory, cover with a sage leaf and sprinkle with salt and pepper.
8. Chop the ham and put it on the baking dish. Sprinkle with cheese and drizzle with liquid orange and butter. Bake in the oven for 10 minutes, then serve hot.

Nutrition:

- Calories: 75 kcal
- Carbs: 0.1 g
- Protein: 13.4 g
- Fat: 1.7 g
- Sugar: 0 g
- Sodium: 253 mg

177. Pork Medallions With Asparagus And Coconut Curry

Preparation Time: 10 minutes

Cooking Time: 15 minutes

Servings: 4–8

Ingredients:

- 1 kg white asparagus
- 500 g carrots
- 2 onions
- 1 red chili pepper
- 40 g butter
- 3–4 tbsp. curry powder
- 250 ml vegetable stock
- 400 ml coconut milk
- 2–3 tbsp. lime juice
- Salt
- Pepper
- 1 tbsp. chopped coriander
- 4 pork medallions (125 g each)
- 2–3 tbsp. oil

Directions:

1. First, peel the asparagus and remove the woody ends, wash well and cut into bite-sized pieces. Then, peel the carrots, wash and cut them into slices. Now, take the onions, remove the skin, and cut them into cubes. Divide the chili in half, take out the seeds, and carefully dice.
2. Put the butter in a pan and heat over medium fire until it has melted.
3. Put the onions and chili in the hot oil and saute until translucent. Add asparagus, carrots and fry everything for 5 minutes, stirring regularly.
4. Pour the curry over it and fry briefly before adding the broth. Set the heat, cover the saucepan and simmer for 10 minutes.
5. Add in the coconut milk and cook for 3 more minutes. Pour in lime juice, salt, and pepper to taste. Sprinkle on 1/2 tbsp. of coriander; stir well.
6. Now, take the meat and season with salt and pepper on both sides. Put the oil in a pan and heat over medium fire.
7. Place the medallions in the hot oil and fry briefly on both sides for about 3–5minutes.
8. Arrange medallions with curry on a plate, garnish with coriander and serve hot.

Nutrition:

- Calories: 432 kcal
- Fat: 12 g
- Carbs: 12 g
- Sugar: 5 g
- Fiber: 3 g
- Protein: 57 g
- Sodium: 566 mg

178. Lamb with Carrot and Brussels Sprouts Spaghetti

Preparation Time: 10 minutes

Cooking Time: 15 minutes

Servings: 4–8

Ingredients:

- 250 g Brussels sprouts
- 300 g carrots
- 5 tbsp. sesame oil
- 3 tbsp. soy sauce
- 1 lime juice
- A Sugar pinch
- Salt
- 600 g loosened saddle of lamb
- Pepper

- 2 tbsp. butter
- 2 tbsp. sesame seeds

Directions:

1. First, preheat the oven to 100ºC.
2. Take the Brussels sprouts, wash, and clean. Then, cut them into strips.
3. For preparing the marinade, place 3 tbsp. of sesame oil together with soy sauce, sugar, salt, and lime juice in a bowl; merge well.
4. Put the vegetable spaghetti in the marinade and let it steep for a moment.
5. In the meantime, flavor the lamb with salt and pepper. Pour the remaining oil into a coated pan and heat on high.
6. Set the meat in the hot oil and sear it on all sides, then put it in the oven and let it cook gently for 10 minutes.
7. After that, melt the butter in the same pan and fry the marinated vegetables for about 3–4 minutes. Arrange on a plate with the sliced lamb and garnish with sesame seeds.

Nutrition:

- Calories: 270 kcal
- Fat: 11 g
- Carbs: 4 g
- Sugar: 1 g
- Fiber: 1 g
- Protein: 39 g
- Sodium: 664 mg

Measurement Conversion Tables

US Dry Volume Measurements	
1/16 tsp.	A dash
1/8 tsp.	A pinch
3 tsp.	1 tbsp.
¼ cup	4 tbsp.
1/3 cup	5 tbsp. + 1 tsp.
½ cup	8 tbsp.
¾ cup	12 tbsp.
1 cup	16 tbsp.
1 pound	16 ounces

US Liquid Volume Measurements	
Eight fluid ounces	1 cup
1 pint = 2 cups	16 fluid ounces
1 quart = 2 pints	4 cups
1 gallon = 4 quarts	16 cups

Conclusion

Diverticulitis is prevalent in the western world. Most of the time, it can be resolved by a temporal change in diet, along with using the right medication.

However, it can be more serious if one encounters some complications. Your doctor will advise you to seek treatment in the hospital if you have complicated diverticulitis; you may have to go through surgery to correct any damage done to the colon.

If you have diverticulitis or have any further questions about this disease, ensure you speak with your doctor as they will know how to treat the disease as well as support your digestive health.

If you were recently diagnosed with diverticulitis, ask your doctor about the food you need and food you should avoid. If you need further guidance, ask your doctor for a dietician you can talk to. You should deal with a professional that has worked with people with diverticulitis.

Also, always be in touch with your doctor regarding your health.

Printed in Great Britain
by Amazon

77758851R10066